Smoking

**Recent Titles in
Q&A Health Guides**

Sexually Transmitted Diseases: Your Questions Answered
Paul Quinn

Mindfulness and Meditation: Your Questions Answered
Blaise Aguirre

Anxiety and Panic Attacks: Your Questions Answered
Daniel Zwillenberg

Substance Abuse: Your Questions Answered
Romeo Vitelli

Eating Disorders: Your Questions Answered
Justine J. Reel

Food Allergies and Sensitivities: Your Questions Answered
Alice C. Richer

Obesity: Your Questions Answered
Christine L. B. Selby

Birth Control: Your Questions Answered
Paul Quinn

Therapy and Counseling: Your Questions Answered
Christine L. B. Selby

Depression: Your Questions Answered
Romeo Vitelli

Food Labels: Your Questions Answered
Barbara A. Brehm

Smoking

Your Questions Answered

Stacy Mintzer Herlihy

Q&A Health Guides

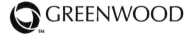

An Imprint of ABC-CLIO, LLC
Santa Barbara, California • Denver, Colorado

Copyright © 2020 by ABC-CLIO, LLC

Library of Congress Cataloging-in-Publication Data

Names: Herlihy, Stacy Mintzer, 1970– author.
Title: Smoking : your questions answered / Stacy Mintzer Herlihy.
Description: Santa Barbara, California : Greenwood, an imprint of ABC-CLIO, LLC,
    [2020] | Series: Q&A health guides | Includes bibliographical references and index.
Identifiers: LCCN 2019046704 (print) | LCCN 2019046705 (ebook) |
    ISBN 9781440864513 (paperback) | ISBN 9781440864520 (ebook)
Subjects: LCSH: Teenagers—Tobacco use—United States. | Smoking—
    United States. | Tobacco use—United States—Prevention.
Classification: LCC HV5745 .H47 2020 (print) | LCC HV5745 (ebook) |
    DDC 613.85—dc23
LC record available at https://lccn.loc.gov/2019046704
LC ebook record available at https://lccn.loc.gov/2019046705

ISBN: 978-1-4408-6451-3 (print)
     978-1-4408-6452-0 (ebook)

24 23 22 21 20   1 2 3 4 5

This book is also available as an eBook.

Greenwood
An Imprint of ABC-CLIO, LLC

ABC-CLIO, LLC
147 Castilian Drive
Santa Barbara, California 93117
www.abc-clio.com

This book is printed on acid-free paper ∞

Manufactured in the United States of America

For Brendan, Serena Jane, and Charlotte Winifred. And for my mom, who died from secondhand smoking.

Contents

Series Foreword   xi

Acknowledgments   xiii

Introduction   xv

Guide to Health Literacy   xvii

Common Misconceptions about Smoking   xxv

Questions and Answers   1

General Information   3

    1. What is tobacco?   3
    2. What is nicotine?   5
    3. What forms of smoking exist?   7
    4. What is vaping?   10
    5. Are there harmful ingredients in cigarettes besides
       tobacco and nicotine?   16
    6. How common is smoking in the United States?   18
    7. How common is smoking worldwide?   21
    8. Why do people begin smoking?   22
    9. How does tobacco get into the body?   25
   10. What is secondhand smoke?   27

11. What is thirdhand smoke? 29
12. Are there any benefits to smoking? 33

Smoking Risks 39

13. What are the short-term risks associated with smoking? 39
14. What does smoking do to the lungs? 41
15. What does smoking do to the heart? 44
16. What does smoking do to the brain? 46
17. Can smoking cause lung cancer? 49
18. Is smoking linked to any other kinds of cancer? 51
19. What other diseases and conditions are linked
    to smoking? 53
20. What role do genetics play in the likelihood that
    negative health effects will result from smoking? 58
21. Will smoking hurt me and the baby if I get pregnant? 60
22. Does smoking lead to the use of other drugs? 62
23. Does chewing tobacco pose any special risks? 64
24. Can secondhand and thirdhand smoke pose health risks? 66
25. Are certain forms of smoking, such as vaping and
    low-tar cigarettes, less dangerous? 68
26. Can smoking kill me? 70

Tobacco Industry and Regulation 73

27. When did we discover the negative effects of smoking? 73
28. Why is smoking legal? 76
29. How is tobacco regulated around the world? 78
30. How big is the tobacco industry? 80
31. How is tobacco advertised? 83

Quitting 87

32. How addictive is smoking? 87
33. What is quitting cold turkey? Is it effective? 89
34. If I'm smoking only one or two cigarettes a day,
    do I really need to quit? 90
35. What over-the-counter methods are there to help
    me quit smoking? 92
36. What kind of professional help is available? 95
37. How can I tell my parents about my need to quit? 97
38. What effects might I experience once I begin quitting? 99
39. How can I help someone I care about quit? 101
40. What can I do to help others in my community
    who smoke? 103

41. What if I start smoking again? 105
42. Is quitting smoking harder than quitting drinking? 107
43. What kinds of new treatments are being developed
    to help people quit? 110
44. How can I become part of the antismoking and
    antivaping movement? 112

Case Studies 115

Glossary 125

Directory of Resources 129

Index 133

Series Foreword

All of us have questions about our health. Is this normal? Should I be doing something differently? Whom should I talk to about my concerns? And our modern world is full of answers. Thanks to the Internet, there's a wealth of information at our fingertips, from forums where people can share their personal experiences to Wikipedia articles to the full text of medical studies. But finding the right information can be an intimidating and difficult task—some sources are written at too high a level, others have been oversimplified, while still others are heavily biased or simply inaccurate.

Q&A Health Guides address the needs of readers who want accurate, concise answers to their health questions, authored by reputable and objective experts and written in clear and easy-to-understand language. This series focuses on the topics that matter most to young adult readers, including various aspects of physical and emotional well-being as well as other components of a healthy lifestyle. These guides will also serve as a valuable tool for parents, school counselors, and others who may need to answer teens' health questions.

All books in the series follow the same format to make finding information quick and easy. Each volume begins with an essay on health literacy and why it is so important when it comes to gathering and evaluating health information. Next, the top five myths and misconceptions that surround the topic are dispelled. The heart of each guide is a collection of questions and answers, organized thematically. A selection of five case studies provides real-world examples to illuminate key concepts. Rounding out each volume are a directory of resources, glossary, and index.

It is our hope that the books in this series will not only provide valuable information but will also help guide readers toward a lifetime of healthy decision making.

Acknowledgments

This book is the result of much hard work and a great deal of passion. It's also the result of tremendous help and support from some truly marvelous people I am most lucky to have in my life. I would like to thank Tish Davidson, Allison Hagood, Melody Butler, Cigal Shaham, Michael Simpson, Tati Piv, Lori Boyle, Elizabeth Faber, Marci Swede, Amy Wambsganss, Renee Liss, Malinda Giannetti, Alice Wasney, Ethel Magal, Catherine Lafuente, Marcia Disbrow, Catherina Becker, Craig Egan, Jody Mullen, Jeannette Ratliff, Ursuyl Kukura-Straw, Diana Austin, Wendy Wilkinson, Miriam Simon Zarovsky, and many others.

I would especially like to thank my gifted editor, Maxine Taylor. Her useful guidance, profound understanding of this subject, thoughtful suggestions, and editorial gifts provided me with the help necessary to shape this important manuscript. I would also like to thank my beloved husband, Brendan Herlihy Jr. His patience, kindness, love, and unending support were invaluable during the writing process. This book is for my adored daughters, Serena Jane and Charlotte Winifred. I hope they face a world where tobacco and nicotine addiction are a thing of the past.

Above all, this book is dedicated to the memory of my late mother, Paula Mintzer. My mom had not smoked for decades. Sadly, she died of emphysema from secondhand smoking. We are all the poorer for her early passing.

Introduction

The use of nicotine and other tobacco products dates back almost to the start of human history. Smoking and nicotine use became a popular worldwide trend several hundred years ago. Today, smoking and the use of tobacco products are quite widespread. In the United States, cigarette smoking is on the wane. The same is true of the percentage of American teenagers who smoke. The percentage of adults who smoke has also decreased. The fifty-plus-year campaign to reduce the percentage of smokers in the United States and many other nations is one of the world's greatest public health accomplishments. At the same time, the number of teens who vape is increasingly on the rise in the United States and across the globe. Smoking and vaping are extremely dangerous activities with potentially serious health consequences. Those who smoke or vape are likely to find themselves risking health problems that include cancer as well as heart disease and the possibility of sudden death. It is imperative for parents and teens today to understand these risks and how best to avoid them.

Educational efforts by government officials and those who are responsible for educating teens and parents alike have been an integral part of antismoking campaigns in prior decades. The modern Internet has enabled both bad information and sources of good, accurate, factual evidence. The Internet has also allowed contemporary myths about tobacco smoking and vaping to spread rapidly. Tobacco companies and those that manufacture vaping products have used the Internet and sources such as text messaging and social media to deliberately target the teenage market. Government officials and teen educators must be prepared to counteract such efforts and help teens find the resources they need to avoid smoking and vaping or quit if they have already started.

The purpose of this book is to help counter such efforts and provide a single, valuable resource that can answer common questions educators, teens, and parents have about all aspects of smoking, vaping, and varied forms of nicotine use. Teens, parents, and educators should look to this book as a starting point that can ideally help foster useful discussion. Studies repeatedly show that most people who are hooked on smoking and nicotine products are young people. The aim of this book is to help all concerned work together to overcome issues related to such products and provide teens with a healthier future.

Guide to Health Literacy

On her 13th birthday, Samantha was diagnosed with type 2 diabetes. She consulted her mom and her aunt, both of whom also have type 2 diabetes, and decided to go with their strategy of managing diabetes by taking insulin. As a result of participating in an after-school program at her middle school that focused on health literacy, she learned that she can help manage the level of glucose in her bloodstream by counting her carbohydrate intake, following a diabetic diet, and exercising regularly. But what exactly should she do? How does she keep track of her carbohydrate intake? What is a diabetic diet? How long should she exercise and what type of exercise should she do? Samantha is a visual learner, so she turned to her favorite source of media, YouTube, to answer these questions. She found videos from individuals around the world sharing their experiences and tips, doctors (or at least people who have "Dr." in their YouTube channel names), government agencies such as the National Institutes of Health, and even video clips from cat lovers who have cats with diabetes. With guidance from the librarian and the health and science teachers at her school, she assessed the credibility of the information in these videos and even compared their suggestions to some of the print resources that she was able to find at her school library. Now, she knows exactly how to count her carbohydrate level, how to prepare and follow a diabetic diet, and how much (and what) exercise is needed daily. She intends to share her findings with her mom and her aunt, and now she wants to create a chart that summarizes what she has learned that she can share with her doctor.

Samantha's experience is not unique. She represents a shift in our society; an individual no longer views himself or herself as a passive recipient of medical care but as an active mediator of his or her own health. However, in this era when any individual can post his or her opinions and experiences with a particular health condition online with just a few clicks or publish a memoir, it is vital that people know how to assess the credibility of health information. Gone are the days when "publishing" health information required intense vetting. The health information landscape is highly saturated, and people have innumerable sources where they can find information about practically any health topic. The sources (whether print, online, or a person) that an individual consults for health information are crucial because the accuracy and trustworthiness of the information can potentially affect his or her overall health. The ability to find, select, assess, and use health information constitutes a type of literacy—health literacy—that everyone must possess.

THE DEFINITION AND PHASES OF HEALTH LITERACY

One of the most popular definitions for health literacy comes from Ratzan and Parker (2000), who describe health literacy as "the degree to which individuals have the capacity to obtain, process, and understand basic health information and services needed to make appropriate health decisions." Recent research has extrapolated health literacy into health literacy bits, further shedding light on the multiple phases and literacy practices that are embedded within the multifaceted concept of health literacy. Although this research has focused primarily on online health information seeking, these health literacy bits are needed to successfully navigate both print and online sources. There are six phases of health information seeking: (1) Information Need Identification and Question Formulation, (2) Information Search, (3) Information Comprehension, (4) Information Assessment, (5) Information Management, and (6) Information Use.

The first phase is the *information need identification and question formulation phase*. In this phase, one needs to be able to develop and refine a range of questions to frame one's search and understand relevant health terms. In the second phase, *information search*, one has to possess appropriate searching skills, such as using proper keywords and correct spelling in search terms, especially when using search engines and databases.

It is also crucial to understand how search engines work (i.e., how search results are derived, what the order of the search results means, how to use the snippets that are provided in the search results list to select websites, and how to determine which listings are ads on a search engine results page). One also has to limit reliance on surface characteristics, such as the design of a website or a book (a website or book that appears to have a lot of information or looks aesthetically pleasant does not necessarily mean it has good information) and language used (a website or book that utilizes jargon, the keywords that one used to conduct the search, or the word "information" does not necessarily indicate it will have good information). The next phase is *information comprehension*, whereby one needs to have the ability to read, comprehend, and recall the information (including textual, numerical, and visual content) one has located from the books and/or online resources.

To assess the credibility of health information (*information assessment* phase), one needs to be able to evaluate information for accuracy, evaluate how current the information is (e.g., when a website was last updated or when a book was published), and evaluate the creators of the source—for example, examine site sponsors or type of sites (.com, .gov, .edu, or .org) or the author of a book (practicing doctor, a celebrity doctor, a patient of a specific disease, etc.) to determine the believability of the person/organization providing the information. Such credibility perceptions tend to become generalized, so they must be frequently reexamined (e.g., the belief that a specific news agency always has credible health information needs continuous vetting). One also needs to evaluate the credibility of the medium (e.g., television, Internet, radio, social media, and book) and evaluate—not just accept without questioning—others' claims regarding the validity of a site, book, or other specific source of information. At this stage, one has to "make sense of information gathered from diverse sources by identifying misconceptions, main and supporting ideas, conflicting information, point of view, and biases" (American Association of School Librarians [AASL], 2009, p. 13) and conclude which sources/information are valid and accurate by using conscious strategies rather than simply using intuitive judgments or "rules of thumb." This phase is the most challenging segment of health information seeking and serves as a determinant of success (or lack thereof) in the information-seeking process. The following section, Sources of Health Information, further explains this phase.

The fifth phase is *information management*, whereby one has to organize information that has been gathered in some manner to ensure easy retrieval and use in the future. The last phase is *information use*, in which one will synthesize information found across various resources, draw conclusions, and locate the answer to his or her original question and/or the content that fulfills the information need. This phase also often involves implementation, such as using the information to solve a health problem; make health-related decisions; identify and engage in behaviors that will help a person to avoid health risks; share the health information found with family members and friends who may benefit from it; and advocate more broadly for personal, family, or community health.

THE IMPORTANCE OF HEALTH LITERACY

The conception of health has moved from a passive view (someone is either well or ill) to one that is more active and process based (someone is working toward preventing or managing disease). Hence, the dominant focus has shifted from doctors and treatments to patients and prevention, resulting in the need to strengthen our ability and confidence (as patients and consumers of health care) to look for, assess, understand, manage, share, adapt, and use health-related information. An individual's health literacy level has been found to predict his or her health status better than age, race, educational attainment, employment status, and income level (National Network of Libraries of Medicine, 2013). Greater health literacy also enables individuals to better communicate with health care providers such as doctors, nutritionists, and therapists, as they can pose more relevant, informed, and useful questions to health care providers. Another added advantage of greater health literacy is better information-seeking skills, not only for health but also in other domains, such as completing assignments for school.

SOURCES OF HEALTH INFORMATION: THE GOOD, THE BAD, AND THE IN-BETWEEN

For generations, doctors, nurses, nutritionists, health coaches, and other health professionals have been the trusted sources of health information. Additionally, researchers have found that young adults, when they have health-related questions, typically turn to a family member who has had firsthand experience with a health condition because of their family member's close proximity and because of their past experience with, and trust in, this individual. Expertise should be a core consideration when consulting a person, website, or book for health information. The credentials and background of the person or author and conflicting interests of the author (and his or her organization) must be checked and validated to ensure the likely credibility of the health information they are conveying. While books often have implied credibility because of the peer-review process involved, self-publishing has challenged this credibility, so qualifications of book authors should also be verified. When it comes to health information, currency of the source must also be examined. When examining health information/studies presented, pay attention to the exhaustiveness of research methods utilized to offer recommendations or conclusions. Small and nondiverse sample size is often—but not always—an indication of reduced credibility. Studies that confuse correlation with causation is another potential issue to watch for. Information seekers must also pay attention to the sponsors of the research studies. For example, if a study is sponsored by manufacturers of drug Y and the study recommends that drug Y is the best treatment to manage or cure a disease, this may indicate a lack of objectivity on the part of the researchers.

The Internet is rapidly becoming one of the main sources of health information. Online forums, news agencies, personal blogs, social media sites, pharmacy sites, and celebrity "doctors" are all offering medical and health information targeted to various types of people in regard to all types of diseases and symptoms. There are professional journalists, citizen journalists, hoaxers, and people paid to write fake health news on various sites that may appear to have a legitimate domain name and may even have authors who claim to have professional credentials, such as an MD. All these sites *may* offer useful information or information that appears to be useful and relevant; however, much of the information may be debatable and may fall into gray areas that require readers to discern credibility, reliability, and biases.

While broad recognition and acceptance of certain media, institutions, and people often serve as the most popular determining factors to assess credibility of health information among young people, keep in mind that there are legitimate Internet sites, databases, and books that publish health information and serve as sources of health information for doctors, other health sites, and members of the public. For example, MedlinePlus (https://medlineplus.gov) has trusted sources on over 975 diseases and conditions and presents the information in easy-to-understand language.

The chart here presents factors to consider when assessing credibility of health information. However, keep in mind that these factors function only as a guide and require continuous updating to keep abreast with the changes in the landscape of health information, information sources, and technologies.

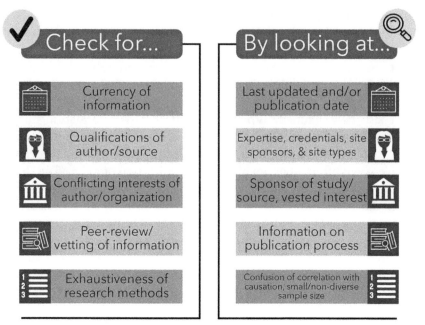

All images from flaticon.com

The chart can serve as a guide; however, approaching a librarian about how one can go about assessing the credibility of both print and online health information is far more effective than using generic checklist-type tools. While librarians are not health experts, they can apply and teach patrons strategies to determine the credibility of health information.

With the prevalence of fake sites and fake resources that appear to be legitimate, it is important to use the following health information assessment tips to verify the health information that one has obtained (St. Jean et al., 2015, p. 151):

- **Don't assume you are right**: Even when you feel very sure about an answer, keep in mind that the answer may not be correct, and it is important to conduct (further) searches to validate the information.
- **Don't assume you are wrong**: You may actually have correct information, even if the information you encounter does not match—that is, you may be right and the resources that you have found may contain false information.
- **Take an open approach**: Maintain a critical stance by not including your preexisting beliefs as keywords (or letting them influence your

choice of keywords) in a search, as this may influence what it is possible to find out.

- **Verify, verify, and verify**: Information found, especially on the Internet, needs to be validated, no matter how the information appears on the site (i.e., regardless of the appearance of the site or the quantity of information that is included).

Health literacy comes with experience navigating health information. Professional sources of health information, such as doctors, health care providers, and health databases, are still the best, but one also has the power to search for health information and then verify it by consulting with these trusted sources and by using the health information assessment tips and guide shared previously.

Mega Subramaniam, PhD
Associate Professor, College of Information
Studies, University of Maryland

REFERENCES AND FURTHER READING

American Association of School Librarians (AASL). (2009). *Standards for the 21st-century learner in action.* Chicago, IL: American Association of School Librarians.

Hilligoss, B., & Rieh, S.-Y. (2008). Developing a unifying framework of credibility assessment: Construct, heuristics, and interaction in context. *Information Processing & Management, 44*(4), 1467–1484.

Kuhlthau, C. C. (1988). Developing a model of the library search process: Cognitive and affective aspects. *Reference Quarterly, 28*(2), 232–242.

National Network of Libraries of Medicine (NNLM). (2013). Health literacy. Bethesda, MD: National Network of Libraries of Medicine. Retrieved from nnlm.gov/outreach/consumer/hlthlit.html

Ratzan, S. C., & Parker, R. M. (2000). Introduction. In C. R. Selden, M. Zorn, S. C. Ratzan, & R. M. Parker (Eds.), *National Library of Medicine current bibliographies in medicine: Health literacy.* NLM Pub. No. CBM 2000–1. Bethesda, MD: National Institutes of Health, U.S. Department of Health and Human Services.

St. Jean, B., Taylor, N. G., Kodama, C., & Subramaniam, M. (February 2017). Assessing the health information source perceptions of tweens using card-sorting exercises. *Journal of Information Science.* Retrieved from http://journals.sagepub.com/doi/abs/10.1177/0165551516687728

St. Jean, B., Subramaniam, M., Taylor, N.G., Follman, R., Kodama, C., & Casciotti, D. (2015). The influence of positive hypothesis testing on youths' online health-related information seeking. *New Library World*, *116*(3/4), 136–154.

Subramaniam, M., St. Jean, B., Taylor, N.G., Kodama, C., Follman, R., & Casciotti, D. (2015). Bit by bit: Using design-based research to improve the health literacy of adolescents. *JMIR Research Protocols*, *4*(2), paper e62. Retrieved from http://www.ncbi.nlm.nih.gov/pmc/articles/PMC4464334/

Valenza, J. (2016, November 26). Truth, truthiness, and triangulation: A news literacy toolkit for a "post-truth" world [Web log]. Retrieved from http://blogs.slj.com/neverendingsearch/2016/11/26/truth-truthiness-triangulation-and-the-librarian-way-a-news-literacy-toolkit-for-a-post-truth-world/

Common Misconceptions
about Smoking

1. THERE ARE NO SHORT-TERM HEALTH
EFFECTS FROM SMOKING

On the surface, smoking would appear to have few, if any, short-term effects. Users pick up a cigarette, and the smoke gets into their lungs. They feel a little relaxed and content as the smoke flows through their veins. Even after a few short puffs, smoking begins to have serious effects. Tobacco starts to change the brain's chemistry immediately after a single cigarette. Even just a few cigarettes can lead to an addiction that the smoker might find hard to shake for many years. The short-term effects of smoking lead to many immediate problems. It starts with the mouth. Smoking stains teeth shades of brown or yellow. It can lead to bad breath and a bad taste in the mouth even when not smoking. Smoke gets on clothing and stays there. When not smoking, the smoke lingers on that favorite cashmere sweater. It makes the best pair of jeans smell badly forever. On a short-term basis, smoking decreases lung capacity. Smokers find it harder to run a simple race or even up a lone flight of stairs. Teens who start to smoke before their lungs are fully developed have stunted lung capacity that cannot be regained. Smoke gets into the respiratory system and makes it harder to take a deep breath. After a round of smoking, the smoker might notice they are developing a cough. Asthma sufferers will have asthma attacks that are both more frequent and more dangerous. Smokers are more susceptible to bronchitis and more likely to get serious infections than peers who do not smoke. The heart rate starts to increase, stressing that muscle and making the heartbeat less efficient. Smoking also has another insidious possibility. Leave that cigarette burning, walk away, and it could set a fire. The number one cause of death from fires is a lit cigarette. Start to smoke, and start a cascade of serious short-term events. You are decreasing your capacity to inhale, stunting the growth of your lungs, staining your favorite clothing, and putting yourself and your loved ones at risk from fire that might engulf your home. For further information on the short-term consequences of smoking, see Question 13.

2. SOCIAL SMOKING IS NOT ADDICTIVE

Hanging out with friends is a favorite pastime. When teens are with friends, they tend to do what they're doing. If peers smoke, chances are that you might bum a cigarette and follow them. Smoking in groups with peers now and then is known as social smoking. Social smoking is when people smoke mostly with their BFFs and not on their own. People might think of themselves as "only" a social smoker or perhaps a "light smoker." These descriptions make the act of smoking feel more comfortable and less dangerous. Just because a person isn't smoking a pack or more a day doesn't mean that social smoking is not addictive. Even a few cigarettes once or twice a week can cause harm. Over time, what seems like only a few smokes can easily become an addiction. For some teens, just a single cigarette a month can bring on an addiction and lead to more smoking as the body experiences nicotine deprivation. Hanging out with peers who smoke means not only exposure to their own smoke. They're also being exposed to secondhand smoke. This can contribute to them becoming addicted to cigarettes and vaping. A few cigarettes now and then or vaping sessions in your own home can also stain walls and other items in the home as part of a process known as thirdhand smoke. Thirdhand smoke leaves a residue of chemicals on all the walls in the room and furniture. Not only is it very hard to remove, it also presents a health hazard. Smoke just four or five cigarettes a week, and the smoker vastly increases their odds of dying compared to those who never light up in the first place. Those who smoke only socially may think that they'll continue to be light smokers forever. They might think it's only a few cigarettes or some vaping now and then and they can stop. However, studies repeatedly show that many people who are light smokers don't stay in that category. Over time, many will find themselves smoking more and more often. On the surface, what felt like a habit they can quit any time starts to quickly become an addiction. Light smoking is just as addictive as heavier smoking and equally dangerous. The good news? Someone who only smokes now and then can find it easier to quit smoking. For the social smoker, now is the time to make a vow to quit smoking and vaping altogether and keep it. For more information, see Question 34.

3. E-CIGS AND VAPING ARE HARMLESS

E-cigs are one of the newest types of nicotine delivery methods. Many teens think that e-cigs and vaping are harmless. Flavors like blueberry and banana split make e-cigs and vaping feel akin to eating a piece of candy or chewing gum. Teens imagine that using e-cigs and vaping in moderate amounts are not dangerous. What many fail to realize is that e-cigs and vaping carry just as many risks as other forms of smoking. In the short term, vaping and the use of e-cigs can lead to serious addiction problems that make it hard to quit smoking both e-cigs and standard cigarettes. In the long run, vaping can also lead to potentially serious and dangerous health effects that may not be readily apparent for months or even years. While vaping and e-cigs are still being studied more extensively right now, it's clear that even greater physical problems from their use may develop over time. It's best to avoid smoking e-cigs and vaping and avoid the potential health risks that can come with them. For more information about this issue, see Questions 4 and 25.

4. QUITTING IS EASY

Quitting smoking seems like the easiest thing ever. The smoker picks up a cigarette, lights the end, inhales a bit, relaxes in the moment, and then puts it down without any care or further thought. Then they pick up another one and do the same thing again and again. Many teens think that they can stop smoking anytime they want. All they have to do is stop using cigarettes and they'll never want to smoke again. On the surface this may seem true and feel accurate. However, as so many smokers have learned over time, it's not remotely that simple. While it may feel as if they can stop smoking cigarettes or vaping, in truth, like many teens they gradually realize that they are unable to shake the habit even if they want to quit. Quitting smoking is not the easy task they thought. In fact, the chemicals in nicotine are some of the most addictive substances ever discovered. When they get into the body, they will alter the body's chemistry. From the very first lit cigarette, the effects of substances such as nicotine and tobacco trigger changes that can be long lasting and terribly difficult to overcome. A smoker may find it easy to quit—only to realize that the cravings have come on strongly. Suddenly the smoker is searching for cigarettes yet again almost against their will. Sure, they can quit smoking in a heartbeat, but they may have to do it again and again and again over a long time in order to be able to finally let it go. See Question 32 for more information.

5. SMOKING ONLY HARMS OLD PEOPLE

The classic image of the damage smoking can cause is an older person with gray hair tethered to an oxygen tank. It is true that certain chronic and fatal diseases like lung cancer and heart disease may take years, if not decades, to develop. These diseases are linked to smoking. It is true they are rarely, if ever, seen in teens. At the same time, smoking has harmful effects that can show up far earlier than many teens think. Damaging effects can be apparent shortly after the smoker begins smoking. According to the World Health Organization, early signs of heart disease and stroke can even be found in adolescents who smoke and vape. Young athletes may notice a decrease in their abilities after smoking for as little as a few weeks. They may find that they are unable to run as fast, jump as high, or last as long on the field before they began smoking. Young women may find themselves staring at unwanted facial wrinkles long before their peers. A teen can quickly develop a smoker's cough that can linger for weeks, if not months, and be difficult to shake off. Such coughs are debilitating and hard to control. Teens may also suffer from depression and other mental health effects as the ingredients in cigarettes and other tobacco products can actually change the brain's chemistry. As adolescents grow, they may find that smoking can alter their physique by stunting their rib cage and reducing their overall lung capacity. More details about exactly how smoking can damage your health can be found in Questions 13–26.

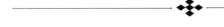

QUESTIONS AND ANSWERS

General Information

I. What is tobacco?

When discussing smoking, it is crucial to understand the terms used. Tobacco or *Nicotiana tabacum Linné* is a plant. Tobacco stimulates the nervous system. The body responds by increasing heart rate and blood pressure. Tobacco also irritates internal tissues and may affect many senses, including your ability to smell and hear. *Nicotiana tabacum Linné* is in nearly all forms of smoking products, including many e-cigs. Although it has become widely popular in much of the world only in the last few centuries, it is believed people have been growing tobacco plants to smoke or for their own use for over five thousand years. Tobacco plants are thought to have been first cultivated in the Americas. Columbus described natives of Cuba who were smoking a plant that was unknown at the time in the rest of the world. He brought it home as a curiosity. The new plant quickly became popular in Europe, where it was widely hailed as a miracle drug that could help everything from insomnia to migraines. As global trade and commerce increased, so did use of tobacco in the rest of the world. Today, we know a great deal more about tobacco, its effects, and how it can lead to serious harm when used over time.

Tobacco plants may grow more than six feet tall when reaching their full growth and have a sticky feel when touched. Tobacco plants are coated with nicotine. Nicotine is the primary substance that makes the tobacco plant different from other plants. The tobacco product that is cultivated today for commercial use has many parts. Five petals in the center come in varied colors. As it continues to grow, the plant bears seeds known as tobacco fruit. Perhaps the most notable part of the plant are the leaves. They may easily grow over a foot long and nearly a foot wide. Tobacco leaves come in many kinds of shapes that vary from variety to variety, including heart shaped and egg shaped. These are bright green when ready to be harvested. Tobacco is a widely grown plant. In fact, it is the world's single-most widely grown nonfood crop. There are more than seventy varieties commonly in production at any given time. Major tobacco-producing countries include the United States, China, Brazil, and India. It is commonly grown in other places as diverse as Philippines and South Africa. Each year, growers produce about eight million tons of tobacco for harvest. American farmers grow about two hundred thousand tons of tobacco. Three states, Georgia, Kentucky, and North Carolina, produce about 80 percent of the American tobacco crop.

Plants intended for commercial sale are first grown in dedicated indoor beds known as hotbeds. Tobacco farmers create tobacco hotbeds that are grown directly from seeds. Seeds are allowed to grow for about eight weeks until they can withstand problems outdoors such as insects and bad weather. After this time, farmers snip off the top of the plant. This makes sure that the plant's energy is devoted entirely to growing the leaves farmers want instead of flowers that will not yield nicotine they need to make tobacco products. Plants are then removed to the tobacco fields for further growth. Growers want to have tobacco leaves that are long and thick because they make the ideal tobacco end product. The plants stay in the fields for about four months, until they are typically harvested by hand on small farms in less developed nations and by machinery on larger farms in more developed countries.

Fertilizer is frequently used to help the plant's leaves grow even larger. Special care must be taken when growing tobacco as it can easily deplete many soil nutrients in a short time. While this is not as much of a problem in places such as the United States, where modern farming techniques are frequently used and farmers get subsidies from the government, it can be a serious issue in many low-income countries. Production is often done by small-scale producers with perhaps only a few acres under cultivation. The reduction in nutrients can eat into the farmer's profits. It can also leave the soil unsuitable for any other crop for several years. A large tobacco buying company in such low-income countries can set prices low for wholesale products. This makes it even harder for farmers to earn a profit. Many farmers in low-income countries put aside crops that can be used as food in favor of growing tobacco for a slim profit that may barely feed their family. Such farms may require help from all members of the family to bring the crop to market. Children as young as seven assist their families in growing tobacco. Lots of pesticides are often used to increase yield and decrease loss from agricultural pests. Early exposure to pesticides may increase a young child's long-term risk of cancer and cause other health issues, including developmental delays.

Once leaves are harvested, they must be dried in order to make them ready to turn them into products for the market. Leaves are dried to remove moisture and aged to make them more palatable to the smoker. Various methods are used to dry or cure the tobacco leaves. In general, tobacco leaves are kept in a barn and dried by air. Tobacco can also be dried by a slow burning fire. In parts of the world, where it is very sunny, the leaves are left outdoors to dry in the sun. After the tobacco leaves have been harvested and dried, they are then gathered into bundles. Bundles are aged for anywhere from a year to three years. Most tobacco farmers sell the finished product to a tobacco company once their product is dried.

2. What is nicotine?

Tobacco products have many components. Experts estimate that there are about four thousand chemicals in a single cigarette, cigar, or bit of snuff. Chemicals found in all tobacco products, including many kinds of e-cigs, are known to have extremely harmful effects. Nicotine, found in tobacco leaves, is a crucial substance that is used in almost every single form of smoking, including many forms of e-cigs. Jean Nicot, who gave his name to the quintessential product, was the French ambassador to Portugal. He is credited with bringing the snuff form of tobacco to the French court in the 1600s. People of all backgrounds and classes used nicotine in varied forms at court, where it then spread to many parts of Europe. While the tobacco plant was originally called "nicotina," the term has since been used to refer to the chemical in the plant rather than the entire plant. When looked at in direct sunlight, nicotine is just a colorless liquid. Light it with a match, and watch as it turns a muddy brown.

Research on the properties of nicotine continues. Nicotine is known to be a very highly addictive substance that can lead to lifelong addiction even after a single cigarette. Companies that sell smoking and tobacco products want customers to crave their products and serve as a ready market. It's also one of the many reasons why so many people find it very hard to quit smoking or why they attempt to quit and fail multiple times. People can absorb nicotine in lots of different ways, including chewing tobacco and e-cigs. Those who smoke the chemical inhale its nicotine directly into their lungs. If tobacco is chewed or sniffed, it gets into the body via the mucous membranes present in the mouth and nose. Even touching nicotine can cause it to get into the skin immediately. From there, it can spread very quickly. When discussing nicotine, it's helpful to keep two terms in mind. "Pharmacokinetics" is used to refer to what the body does to any substance the body may encounter. "Pharmacodynamics" refers to what the substance does to the body. While nicotine gets into the brain in as little as eight seconds, it can linger for many hours until finally excreted, changing the chemistry of the brain and making it respond to the presence of nicotine directly.

Nicotine is actually both a stimulant that speeds up the body's metabolism and a sedative that slows it down. This is because nicotine acts directly on the adrenal glands and brings a rush of a stimulant called adrenaline. The pancreas releases less insulin in response to nicotine. A smoker's blood pressure goes up along with their heart rate. However, after it gets into the brain, it can stimulate the brain to release certain chemicals, including beta-endorphin, serotonin, and opioids. These are substances that may reduce anxiety and make the user feel sleepier. Nicotine also causes a chemical in the brain called dopamine to be released, making users feel a sense of pleasure. The effect is comparable to using "harder" drugs such as cocaine and heroin.

The substance can create a deficit that can easily and quickly lead to addiction. Tolerance means that as the user continues to use nicotine, it takes longer and longer for them to experience the effects of nicotine. A person may smoke a cigarette and feel an intense rush of stimulation in the morning from the nicotine. As the day continues and they continue to smoke, the effects may not be as noticeable. This is why many smokers will speak about how their very first smoke of the day is the most important to them. When not smoking at night, the body's levels of nicotine fall because the smoker is not getting up every so often during the night to smoke and keep up the body's level of nicotine. The first smoke of the day is a fresh hit of nicotine. Even as they continues to take smoke breaks throughout the rest of the day, the feeling will not be as deep. The amount of nicotine acting on the brain can dissipate in a few minutes. Over time, it can take more and more nicotine to achieve the desired result and help the user continue that first pleasing hit. This is one of many reasons why nicotine in any form, including e-cigs, is so addictive. It enters the body quickly and then leaves in a few hours, leaving the smoker wanting yet more each day and often desperate to get it again and again and again. As nicotine is removed, the user starts to feel a sense of decreased pleasure and increased anxiety. Many smokers feel the need to keep a certain level of nicotine all day long, or they simply don't feel good. Nicotine can ultimately change the body's fundamental chemistry.

3. What forms of smoking exist?

Many forms of tobacco delivery systems can be purchased and/or created. In general there are several basic ways to smoke, use, or inhale tobacco. Such methods include cigarettes, cigars, dissolvable tobacco, e-cigs, hookahs, kreteks, and pipes. Each form uses a different method to deliver tobacco to the body. Some methods have been used for centuries, while others are of relatively recent origin.

Cigarettes

The cigarette is the most widely used form of tobacco. A cigarette consists of a cylinder containing tobacco that is either ground or shredded. The ground tobacco is then wrapped around paper or other material similar to paper. In many Asian countries, cigarettes are wrapped in a tembhurni leaf native to the area. These are known as bidis and are commonly seen in many Asian nations. Cigarettes are made by companies and have filters at one end while the other is smoked. The filters are designed to trap some of the harmful chemicals in the cigarette and prevent them from getting into the smoker's lungs.

Cigars and Cigarillos

Cigars and cigarillos differ somewhat from cigarettes. Like cigarettes, these are rolled tubes of tobacco. However, unlike cigarettes, the tobacco is wrapped in leaves and then fermented before being formed into cigars. Cigar use dates back centuries in the Americas. A typical cigar will last longer and take longer to smoke than a cigarette. They are larger, long, and do not contain a filter. Cigarillos are also known as little cigars. These are quite similar in size to cigarettes. They are often flavored and may be sold as a single product or in packages. Both cigars and cigarillos contain more tobacco than cigarettes. While some people choose to inhale the smoke, many do not. Smokers who do not inhale receive tobacco via the mouth.

Dissolvable Tobacco

A relatively new addition to the tobacco delivery system market, dissolvable tobacco is compressed tobacco that has been heavily processed. The tobacco is then turned into small, shaped pellets that can be directly dissolved on the mouth or tongue. Dissolvable tobacco can be found in many forms, including shapes such as toothpicks, mint-flavored gum-like pieces, and small strips. These differ from many other delivery methods because they do not generate smoke. Unlike tobacco chews, they do not require the user to spit out the used tobacco. While marketed as a method to help people quit smoking, many smokers actually use them as part of their smoking routine along with other forms of tobacco products.

Hookahs

Dating back over five hundred years ago, a hookah is an ancient smoking delivery method. It is commonly used in Asia and the Middle East as well as hookah bars in contemporary Europe. Hookah types and components generally consist of a few basic parts. The pipe attaches to a chamber filled with smoke. A hookah also has a bowl and a large or small hose that can be made from varied materials, including birch and rubber. Users take in the smoke via a form of tobacco that has been specially designed for it. As it heats up, smoke from the bowl passes through water and into the pipe. Smokers inhale the smoke through a mouthpiece that is attached to the pipe. Users often add flavorings to the liquid in addition to the flavor from the tobacco. Unlike cigarettes, hookahs do not have any filters, so the user directly gets full exposure to tobacco.

Kreteks or Clove Cigarettes

Kreteks are commonly known as clove cigarettes in much of the world. Originating in Indonesia over a hundred years ago, clove cigarettes are seen in many countries. Like cigarettes, they consist of a long cylindrical tube that the user smokes. Kreteks are filled with a mixture of tobacco and cloves. The tobacco is ground and so are the cloves. Clove oil is typically added to the Kreteks. A standard clove cigarette will be about 30 percent cloves by weight. Additional spices may also be added to the cigarettes such as licorice and anise. The clove cigarette may or may not have a filter at one end. As of September 22, 2009, it is no longer legal to sell these cigarettes in the United States. They are sold legally in other nations.

Pipes

Perhaps the oldest of all smoking delivery methods, the pipe has been in use across the globe for centuries. Pipes are made of three parts. A bowl sticks out at one end. This is where the tobacco is kept. A thin tube or shank is at one end and is used to draw the smoke up the chamber. A mouthpiece is attached at the other end. Pipes are most commonly made of wood. Other materials such as porcelain and corncobs have also been used. Unlike many forms of cigarettes, pipes do not have a filter that can help remove some of the most dangerous chemicals.

Smokeless Tobacco

While most forms of tobacco are lit and then smoked, many users also use smokeless tobacco. Smokeless tobacco goes by many names. It is often called chewing tobacco to distinguish it from regular smoking tobacco. Some people call it spitting tobacco because it is spit from the mouth. Historically, smoking tobacco has also been known as snuff. Snuff is finely powdered tobacco that can be sold in dry or liquid form. This kind of tobacco can also be sniffed. Most people, however, choose to use it by placing it in their cheeks. Users can chew the tobacco or simply suck on it and then spit or swallow the substance.

Electronic Cigarettes or E-Cigs

Electronic cigarettes, also known as e-cigs, are a relatively modern development. They can look like standard cigarettes. Many users rely on a specific delivery method consisting of a small, battery-powered, stand-alone device. People buy a delivery system with a heated coil that vaporizes a solution and then turns it into an aerosol mist. Inhaling this mist is called vaping. People inhale the mist via a device that looks very similar to a cigarette but can be used again and again. Unlike cigarettes, e-cigs do not contain tobacco. They do contain nicotine. Many e-cigs also contain liquefied flavorings in the form of a mist such as chocolate, cherry, and mint that can be changed according to the user's preferences. Electronic cigarettes also have a substance called propylene glycol. This liquid has long been added to many products such as food and cosmetics in order to help the products retain moisture. While often presented as a risk-free alternative to smoking, e-cigs carry many dangers. E-cigs are discussed in more detail in the next question.

4. What is vaping?

An e-cig is also known as an electronic cigarette. Electronic cigarettes have become quite popular in recent years, particularly among teenagers. About one in five teenage boys use e-cigs, while about one in six girls do so. Officials at the Centers for Disease Control and Prevention (CDC) have asserted that more and more teens are being hooked on vaping. Vaping is actually largely responsible for much teen exposure to nicotine and tobacco today. Major cigarette companies such as Philip Morris own shares in companies like JUUL that market e-cigs directly to teens. With an estimated market of roughly $2.5 billion in revenues, e-cigs are big business and rapidly becoming an even bigger business. In the recent past, e-cig use has increased nearly a thousandfold among teens. Many towns have shops that specialize in selling these types of cigarettes only and the vaping equipment that goes with them.

According to repeated polling, a significant percentage of teens and even their parents tend to believe these forms of cigarettes are not only far safer than other types of smoking but also totally safe to consume. Very few understand the true dangers of this newest form of smoking. E-cigs now come in many types besides the standard cigarette. People who want to start vaping or have already done so can find several types of smoking devices that are just like their standard smoking counterparts, including e-hookahs, e-cigars, e-pens, JUUL, and e-pipes. All of these forms of e-cigarettes are grouped together under what are known as electronic nicotine delivery systems (ENDS). ENDS are quite similar to other types of smoking. While an e-cig and an e-pen may extremely seem different on the surface, in fact each type of electronic smoking delivery method differs only slightly in form.

Contrary to common beliefs, all forms of e-cigs have known health risks. Those who have never seen one in person may be curious about what they look like. In fact, all forms of ENDS also have certain parts in common that differentiate them from standard types of traditional smoking methods. The Food and Drug Administration (FDA) has taken a close look at the creation and advertising of e-cigs. Officials at the FDA have settled on a formal definition of e-cigarettes as a method that allows users to inhale an aerosol or a spray of very small liquid particles. The aerosol in the liquid that is used in e-cigs generally contains nicotine, but some e-cigs do not. The aerosol may also contain additional substances that are not always listed for the user. E-cigs fundamentally differ from other forms of cigarettes in that they have two components not found in traditional forms of cigarettes. Users of e-cig units first buy a basic product they will use over and again. This is the base that contains a battery that pairs with the e-cig. Unlike cigarettes, e-cigs also use some indirect form of heating to create the smoke such as heated metal coil. This is in contrast to the direct smoke-producing flame used to light the standard modern cigarette. When the battery is turned on, the liquid starts to heat up. At this point, the process of using the machine can begin. The process is known as vaping. An e-liquid is then heated in the base of the e-cig. It forms a vapor that users inhale. While some liquids for use in vaping actually have little taste or flavor, many e-liquids have additional additives that are widely anticipated and form much of the attraction of this kind of smoking. These additives are designed to resemble flavors not found in standard cigarettes. They mimic flavors that many young children really like, such as chocolate and almonds or cherries and lime. Many teens who vape do so because they liked the tremendous variety of flavors that are available. Roughly 80 percent of all teens who choose to vape choose vaping liquids with at least one added flavor.

Another form of e-cigs is what is known as JUUL. JUULing, as it has rapidly become known by teens, has seen a huge surge of popularity in the last several years. The sleek design of the mechanism is another reason why so many teens like them. They can be fit into a backpack or purse and have brightly colored pods that look like a flash drive. These are lightweight, portable devices that can be hidden with ease and without a parent knowing the teen is using the e-cig. A single pod, the method used to deliver the nicotine, contains as much nicotine as an entire pack of cigarettes. JUUL has attracted a great deal of attention because it is widely used, can be concealed with ease, resembles a flash drive, and appeals to a wide variety of economic groups and ethnic backgrounds.

Quite a number of teens think that e-cigs are a more modern method of smoking. This leads to the popular belief that such types of cigarettes are somehow safer than standard cigarettes because the harmful chemicals have supposedly been removed. Roughly 60 percent of all teens believe smoking an e-cig is not dangerous as long as the person doesn't smoke every single day. None of these beliefs are true. While e-cigs have increasingly grown in popularity in the last decade, they actually date back nearly a century. Joseph Robinson filed the first patent for e-cigs in 1927. By the 1960s, several additional patents had been filed with the intent of creating an improved version of Robinson's original idea. However, none of these caught on with the American public. Americans preferred to stick with their standard cigarettes as the alternatives were often messy and hard to use while failing to deliver any real taste or flavor. It was not until 2004 that a Chinese national named Hon Lik created the first truly contemporary e-cig. After years of tinkering, he brought his improved and easier version to market. The e-cig he sold was very popular in his home-land China where nicotine has increasingly become part of the culture.

Heavy marketing helped his invention quickly spread to Europe where it also caught on as a form of alternative smoking. In 2007, his version of the e-cig was introduced to the American public at the American Tobacco Expo. Since that time, e-cigs have become especially popular with American teens and the millennial generation. JUUL is so popular that teens often call smoking e-cigs JUULing. American Surgeon General Jerome Adams has "declared electronic cigarette use among America's youth 'an epidemic.'" His office reports one in five American high school seniors have reported being current users of e-cigs. This startling statistic is only expected to grow in the coming years as more and more companies join the e-cig market in hopes of capturing this potentially growing market. Many such companies have made teens aware of these products by ever more aggressive marketing campaigns aimed at both the preteen and teen market. While certain advertisers have chosen to market these devices solely to adults who already smoke, most sellers have largely aimed their efforts at younger buyers, including children still in grade school. They have done so despite the fact that such products cannot be sold to teens in most states. Most teens have seen at least one advertisement for e-cigs.

The CDC found that that more than two-thirds of all teens have seen advertising for e-cigs in places as varied as grocery stores and movies. Manufacturers have spent over a hundred million dollars in yearly advertising in recent years just to increase awareness of e-cigs in this age group. These e-cigs' ads often feature bright colors and the use of design elements that may appeal directly to young children. Finding access to accurate information about this subject can be hard as the products are relatively new on the market. Many adults and teachers know little about them, not having seen them until relatively recently. Many teens like being able to conceal a JUUL pod somewhere a parent or teacher can't find one. Part of the confusion stems from the lack of understanding of exactly what's in e-cigs. Unlike standard cigarettes, e-cigs do not directly contain tobacco. Given how dangerous tobacco is, this leads many teens and even many adults to assume that e-cigs are a healthier alternative to standard cigarettes. While e-cigs and other kinds of electronic delivery devices do not directly contain tobacco, they do contain many other dangerous substances. Just like other forms of smoking, e-cigs start out as a form of tobacco. Growing tobacco is a highly dangerous occupation in and of itself. Land that might otherwise be devoted to nutritious crops such as beans or tomatoes or set aside to grow fodder for animal feed is instead used to grow tobacco. Harvesting tobacco can lead to all sorts of long-term problems for the tobacco field worker.

Dangerous Ingredients

The primary ingredient in e-cigs is nicotine. The nicotine that is extracted from the tobacco is then mixed with some kind of base to form the e-liquid that the end user smokes when they vape. Some companies provide cartridges that claim to be free of nicotine. Repeated studies have shown that companies that sell such e-liquids may not be truthful when making this claim. FDA testing has shown that even cartridges that are marked free of tobacco actually contain measurable amounts when directly tested. Further FDA studies have found that e-liquids that claim to have nicotine often have far greater amounts of nicotine than the amounts listed on the packaging. The newer versions on the market offer even greater exposure to nicotine. Nicotine is not quite as toxic as many of the other chemicals found in standard cigarettes, but it is not a good or desirable ingredient. The argument that because nicotine is not quite as horrible as many chemicals found in e-cigs leads many teens to assume it is safe.

Nicotine is an addictive substance that literally alters the pathways in the brains of users. Chronic use can interfere with a teen's overall brain development, making teens less capable of making mature, adult decisions as they grow up and the prefrontal cortex in the brain reaches full growth. It can also prime the brain to be more accepting of other illicit substances such as cocaine and heroin. Teens and young adults who get pregnant and then vape are putting their babies at risk. Using nicotine via vaping may lead to problems for the baby, such as low birth weight, cognitive impairments, and even fetal deaths. After the baby is born, any exposure to nicotine may increase the risk of SIDS, or sudden infant death syndrome. Teens who use nicotine products of their own may also suffer lasting impairments as they march toward adulthood. Teens tend to be more susceptible than adults to nicotine addiction. As teens vape and increase their exposure to nicotine, they may struggle to break free of the addiction for many years. A 2013 study from the American Society of Cell Biology found that users of e-cigs also had a higher rate of heart disease than their peers.

Nicotine is not the only chemical of concern in e-cigs. The e-liquids may seem completely safe, but they are not. Flavors like Bananas Foster, rainbow candy, and kiwi watermelon seem almost wholesome. Despite the misleading names, in truth such liquids are often far more dangerous than advertised. Researchers at the Harvard T.H. Chan School of Public Health tested fifty-one types of e-liquids. They were looking for the presence of three potentially dangerous chemicals. They found a chemical called diacetyl in 75 percent of all samples. Diacetyl first came to prominence as it sickened microwave popcorn factory workers. When inhaled, the chemical causes a chronic lung disease that damages the lungs and can take years off a person's life. E-liquids are also known to have many other dangerous chemicals. When the coil heats up the liquid, users inhale many toxic chemicals, including formaldehyde and acetaldehyde. These chemicals have been directly linked to cancer. A study in the journal *Environmental Research* found that e-liquids also contained dangerous chemicals when they were not heated. Researchers found alarming levels of nickel, chromium, and manganese. Such chemicals are also known to cause cancer.

Heating e-liquids can create additional problems. Compounds known as volatile organic compounds (VOCs) are found in certain products commonly found in most households including paint thinner, liquid insect pest products, and furniture polish. These products are often used by some teens who are looking for a quick high. VOCs are dangerous for many reasons. They are known to cause short-term problems such as headaches and trouble breathing. Long-term studies have linked them with many kinds of cancers. A report in the journal *Pediatrics* found much greater levels of VOCs in teens who vaped versus those who did not. Toxins such as acrolein that can affect the heart and acrylamide that can irritate the skin and is linked to cancer were discovered in vaping, leading doctors to suggest that even higher levels of such problematic chemicals could accumulate in teens as they continue to vape.

Other Behaviors

Some parents believe that teens who use e-cigs will not use other forms of tobacco or other dangerous substances such as alcohol. Studies have indicated that teens who currently use only e-cigs are actually more likely to use standard cigs in the future. They may get addicted to the sensation of smoking nicotine and want to seek out additional ways to smoke it. Of those high school students who use tobacco products in any form, more people smoke both e-cigarettes and other forms of tobacco products than those who simply use e-cigarettes. Rather than reducing their total consumption of varied forms of tobacco products, users spend even more time being exposed to nicotine, tobacco, and other forms of dangerous chemicals found in different types of smoking. They are also more likely to use other dangerous substances like alcohol and use such substances to a dangerous degree. Some people believe that using e-cigs can help them quit smoking. Indeed, some companies market their e-cigs as a smoking cessation product. However, despite such claims, there's no evidence that those who use e-cigs find it easier to quit smoking in the long term. A study in *the Lancet* found that e-cig users were actually less likely to stop smoking than their peers.

Bodily Harm

In addition to containing harmful chemicals, e-cigs have been directly shown to harm many body parts. Irfan Rahman is a toxicologist at University of Rochester. He and his team of experts found that the smoke found in vaping can lead to mouth problems such as gum disease. Rahman and his team also found that the vapors from e-cigs may impede wound healing. Additional studies have also found that teens who smoke may develop what is known as the smoker's cough and find it hard to catch their breath just like those who use tobacco. A chronic cough can ultimately damage the lungs and lead to a condition known as bronchitis. When vapors heat up the e-liquids even further, as part of a process known as dripping, the results may be even more dangerous. As the liquids are subject to such high heat, they may undergo a transformation that increases the concentration of dangerous chemicals found in the smoke even further.

Simply keeping e-cigs on hand can also cause problems. Young children may be tempted by the colorful packaging and the pleasing flavors they see. They may decide to try the e-liquid for themselves and get very sick. Vapers may also accidentally get the e-liquids on their flesh or ingest the liquid directly. Nicotine poisoning can happen when large doses of e-liquids are ingested. Nicotine poisoning can lead to serious health consequences such as breathing problems, seizures, and even death. A pet can swallow the e-liquid and get sick.

While on the surface, e-cigs may feel like a modern, safe alternative to traditional forms of smoking, in practice nothing could be more inaccurate. E-cigs are harmful products with potentially very dangerous side effects for the user and everyone around them.

5. Are there harmful ingredients in cigarettes besides tobacco and nicotine?

When people smoke, they actually inhale over four thousand separate substances. According to the American Cancer Society, seventy of the chemicals found in cigarette smoke have been directly shown to cause cancer. Teens know that cigarettes contain tobacco and nicotine; chemicals have been linked to health problems ranging from a minor cough to many types of cancers. While tobacco and nicotine are the major cause of serious health issues, there are many other equally harmful ingredients in cigarettes. Such ingredients can cause immediate physical problems such as shortness of breath. In the longer term, they can lead to chronic health issues like emphysema and cancer that lead to a shorter life span and unwanted side effects.

In one sense, anything in large-enough amounts is toxic. Ingest too much water and you drown. One of the most troubling things about the ingredients in cigarettes is just how many substances they contain that are incredibly dangerous even in very tiny amounts. A few puffs and the smoker drags material in the lungs that have been linked with diseases ranging from leukemia to heart disease. Some of the chemical compounds found in cigarette smoke are used to clean bathrooms and preserve dead bodies. Many such chemicals are not only present when the tobacco is harvested. In the process of creating cigarettes and other tobacco products, manufacturers add additional toxic chemicals. While the amounts are fairly low, as the smoker continues to smoke, such dangerous toxins start to accumulate and continue to stay in a smoker's body for years. Smoking just a pack a week can quickly lead to a really sore throat and shortness of breath. Those who smoke for years may ultimately be risking many health problems.

Elemental Dangers

The body contains chemicals that sound dangerous. In such minute amounts, they do not pose a health threat. For example, the body produces formaldehyde. It is also found in foods like pears and will not pose any harm. However, some of the most harmful chemicals in cigarette smoke are elements that are highly dangerous even in small doses.

The elements that are found in toxic quantities in tobacco include the following:

- Arsenic
- Benzene
- Cadmium
- Chromium
- Lead
- Nickel
- Uranium

Arsenic is an element that has long been known to have deleterious effects. It is used to help fertilize tobacco in the fields. The International Agency for Research on Cancer classifies arsenic as a carcinogen. Experts believe arsenic is linked to many kinds of cancers, including skin cancer and kidney cancer. Benzene is a toxic substance that can be found anywhere there's cigarette smoke. Even small amounts can trigger health problems. Studies indicate that it is particularly unsafe to your bone marrow. Over time benzene can cause bone marrow problems that may include exhausting anemia as a result of low red blood cell counts and life-threatening leukemia. Cadmium and chromium are two more of the most hazardous chemicals found in cigarettes. A bluish white metal, cadmium is found in the earth's crust. Today, it's mostly used to make batteries. Breathe in the cadmium found in cigarette smoke as a result of the manufacturing process. It will damage your lungs and hurt your kidneys. According to the federal agency known as the Agency for Toxic Substances and Disease Registry, over time smokers accumulate twice as much cadmium as those who do not smoke, putting them at risk from many health problems, including kidney disease. Cadmium lingers in the air and may be inhaled by nonsmoke. Another metal found in cigarette smoke is chromium. While often found in trace amounts in many foods, in the large amounts found in cigarette smoke, chromium has been linked to heart disease and many cancers. Lead and nickel are also products of smoking. Lead is an incredibly toxic element. In young children, it has been shown to lower a kid's IQ and decrease motor skills. One of the most dangerous aspects of lead is that it can easily get into all of the person's bodily systems. Lead is also not easily excreted. Over time, lead levels will stay in the body and continue to increase if not removed. A pregnant woman who smokes endangers not only her own life but also the life of her developing fetus. The same is true of nickel. Nickel can also damage the baby as the woman smokes. Uranium is one of the most dangerous substances ever discovered. Even in small doses, it has been directly linked with serious health effects. Every single time a smoker smokes, they bring uranium directly into their lungs.

Other Harmful Substances

Many other harmful substances are found in tobacco smoke:

• Carbon monoxide
• Hydrogen cyanide
• Nitrosamines
• Polycyclic aromatic hydrocarbons (PAHs)

Carbon monoxide is produced in the body in very low qualities. A colorless, odorless gas, carbon monoxide is responsible for thousands of cases of poisoning each year. The carbon monoxide found in cigarettes in dangerously high levels can lead to problems including an increased pulse that can ultimately lead to heart disease. Hydrogen cyanide, while colorless and odorless, is incredibly poisonous. It is one of the nearly four hundred additives approved for use in cigarettes by the American government. Zyklon B, as hydrogen cyanide was called during World War II, was used by the Nazis in mobile vans as part of their plans to murder millions of Jews and other innocent victims. In small amounts, it can cause headaches and other minor physical issues. Over time, it can also make it harder for smokers to breathe. Tobacco-specific nitrosamines have been linked to many types of deadly cancers, including cancers of the esophagus and the lungs. PAHs are chemical compounds. They are produced when organic matter is burned. PAHs have been linked to many problems in smokers, including osteoporosis where the body's bones start to break down and develop holes.

6. How common is smoking in the United States?

Over the past several decades, tobacco use in the United States has been steadily declining. According to the CDC, in the mid-1960s, about 40 percent of all American adults were smokers. Today, only about 16 percent of Americans smoke. Health officials hope to see this percentage continue to drop as more and more people become aware of the dangers of smoking. At the same time, the use of vaping and e-cigs is up sharply. More than one in three teens report engaging in this form of smoking.

In the United States, tobacco use varies according to several factors. Men are more likely to be smokers. The gap between male and female tobacco use has been declining in younger people. Today, fewer men are choosing to start smoking, while the percentage of female smokers has remained steady. For both sexes in the United States, the percentage of people between the ages of eighteen and twenty-four who smoke is about 13 percent. Different parts of the United States have different rates of smoking as a percentage of the population. Utah has the lowest percentage of smokers at 12 percent. Kentucky and West Virginia have the highest per capita number of smokers. About 30 percent of adults in both states smoke. American smoking rates can be also grouped by percentage of the population according to larger regions. About 25 percent of people who live in the Midwest and the South are smokers. Smoking rates are about five percentage points lower in the Northeast and along the states of the West Coast. Smokers in the South and Midwest are also more likely to use several forms of tobacco products such as snuff and cigarettes. Young adults in rural areas tend to start smoking at an earlier age than their more urban and suburban counterparts. Adolescents in rural areas are also more likely to smoke on a daily basis. Children are also more likely to be exposed to smoking in enclosed spaces in rural areas than in suburban parts of the country. In addition, children in rural areas are one-third more likely to have at least one parent who smokes than children growing up in urban areas.

Contemporary American smokers are concentrated largely in a single area. Truth Initiative®, the largest American nonprofit public health organization dedicated to fighting smoking, calls this region Tobacco Nation. These twelve states stretch from Alabama to Michigan and include a large swath of the Midwest and Deep South. Young people start smoking here at a much higher rate than the rest of the country and indeed many other parts of the world. This part of America has the world's fifth-highest adult smoking rate. The number of adult smokers here lags behind only China, Indonesia, the Philippines, and Ukraine. If the region were an independent nation, the number of young smokers would put it in fourth place worldwide. Several policies have contributed to the large number of smokers in this part of the country. Such factors include lower tobacco taxes and fewer laws banning smoking in workplaces and restaurants. Unlike many other parts of the country, many parts of Tobacco Nation do not forbid the purchase of tobacco to people under twenty-one.

Outside of Tobacco Nation, smoking in the United States also varies in other ways. The percentage of Americans who smoke was greatest among those who have only a high school diploma. About a third of all people with a GED smoke compared with only about 4 percent of those with a graduate degree. Those who have an income below the poverty line are also twice as likely to smoke as those with an income above it. Ethnic and racial differences are also common. Smoking rates are highest in those who identify as American Indians/Alaska Natives. This may be attributed to many factors. Tobacco smoking has a role in many traditional Native American ceremonies. Buying tobacco is also less costly on tribal lands as it is not subject to certain taxes. Among ethnic groups, tobacco use tends to be lowest in those of non-Hispanic Asian heritage. Smoking is also higher than average in certain other groups. Military veterans and active members tend to have higher rates of smoking than those who have never served in the military in any capacity. Rates are particularly high for those who are actively deployed. Smoking rates are also high for Americans who are part of the lesbian, gay, bisexual, and transgender (LGBT) communities. About 35 percent of all trans individuals are smokers. Smoking is also higher for those Americans who are living with HIV. People who suffer from mental illness and those who have a disability are also far more likely to smoke than the general population. Some of the highest rates of smoking can be found in adults who have a mental health condition and live below the poverty rate. About half of all such people are smokers. Other American groups with higher than average rates of smoking include people with a history of homelessness and those with a prior criminal record.

Vaping and the use of e-cigs tend to be more common among white people and those with higher incomes. A study in *Nicotine & Tobacco Research* "found non-Hispanic white smokers were nearly four times more likely to switch exclusively to vaping than their non-Hispanic black or Hispanic counterparts, while higher-income smokers were twice as likely as lower-income smokers to switch. The researchers also found Hispanic and black smokers were twice as likely to believe e-cigarettes were more harmful than cigarettes, compared to white smokers." The study also found, "Non-Hispanic black smokers were 73 percent less likely, and Hispanic smokers were 74 percent less likely to exclusively switch to e-cigarettes than non-Hispanic white smokers. Smokers with incomes below the federal poverty line were 52 percent less likely to make the switch than smokers whose incomes were at least double the federal poverty line." Low-income participants and Hispanics and blacks were also more likely to have a positive view of tobacco use.

7. How common is smoking worldwide?

Worldwide, the total number of smokers is more than a billion people. Smoking rates vary greatly by country. In some countries, their patterns of smoking are highly similar to that of the United States. Other countries have a vastly different population of tobacco users. Just as health officials in America have engaged in a concerted effort to publicize the dangers of smoking, so too have health officials done the same in countries such as the United Kingdom. Such efforts have paid off. In Australia, for example, the percent of smokers as a percent of the population has declined from about 28 percent in 1989 to about 18 percent today. In the United Kingdom, thanks to the efforts of antismoking campaigns, only about 16 percent of the population smokes. Just like their American counterparts, those who smoke tend to have lower incomes and less education. In many countries, smoking remains a largely male activity. In many European nations, like in the United States, smoking rates are also on the rise by young women while declining in young men. Vaping and e-cig use are on the rise in a number of countries, including the United Kingdom, Japan, Sweden, Italy, India, and China.

In less developed nations, the number of smokers per capita is also increasing. Many factors have contributed to this increase. Tobacco companies have seized on relatively lax tobacco advertising laws to target countries such as India and China. China alone has 350 million smokers, helping to offset the loss of smokers in other parts of the world. The Chinese market for cigarettes is so large because the Chinese use more cigarettes than all other lower- and middle-income countries combined. The lion's share of the rest of the market is spread out between several countries. According to World Health Organization's Officials, about two-thirds of all smokers reside in one of the following ten countries: China, India, the Russian Federation, Indonesia, the United States, Japan, Brazil, Bangladesh, Germany, and Turkey. Several other countries also have relatively high per capita cigarette consumption. Smoking is common in many Eastern European countries such as Belarus and Macedonia. Many smokers in this area not only smoke. They also smoke many cigarettes each day.

States in many nations in this area report smoking rates that exceed two thousand cigarettes per person per year. In Egypt about 40 percent of all men smoke, while only 2 percent of women do. While smoking tobacco is often seen as a traditional male activity, some companies are increasingly aiming their efforts at women. Smoking is portrayed as a glamorous activity and linked to female equality. The number of female smokers may be underestimated. This is because in large part smoking is not considered a socially acceptable activity in countries such as South Korea. The highest growth rate in the cigarette market has been in an area called the Eastern Mediterranean Region. Comprising nation-states ranging from Afghanistan to Yemen, this area has proven fertile ground for tobacco advertising. In countries such as Jordan, Saudi Arabia, and Lebanon, about a third of all men smoke, while about 10 percent of all women use tobacco. Many nations have responded to the issue of smoking among young people by implementing laws attempting to control tobacco use among teenagers. In many nations across the globe from Angola to France to Brazil, it is illegal to sell tobacco products to anyone under eighteen. Many other nations, including Kuwait and Honduras, prohibit the sale of tobacco to anyone under twenty-one.

Smoking in other parts of the world is likely to continue to rise in all age groups, including teens. Tobacco companies hope to offset the decline in smoking in other places by targeting other communities. They also hope to bring in new clients via vaping and e-cigs.

8. Why do people begin smoking?

The dangers of smoking have been known for centuries. From the very first, it was clear that tobacco posed dangers. Early reports of problems such as chronic coughs and problems with breathing began to appear in many accounts by Europeans and Americans. It was not until large-scale scientific studies began that the precise dangers were confirmed. Active antismoking campaigns have been in place for several decades since that time. And yet people still start smoking. Many people start smoking in their teens. At this point in life, a person's ability to reason is not yet fully developed. If you see someone smoking, you might wonder why they began. If you personally choose to smoke, you might not be fully aware how it all started. The answer is sometimes very complicated and sometimes quite simple. Many factors influence the decision to begin smoking. For some, a single factor such as having a mom who smokes may be enough to convince a young woman to do likewise. Others may smoke because of subtle encouragement such as advertising, peers who smoke, and laws that make it easy for them to buy smoking products legally at an early age.

Advertising

One reason why people start smoking is the profound influence of advertising. Tobacco companies spend over $8 billion yearly advertising their products to the public. Officials have made efforts to combat the influence of such funding and try to persuade people to quit. In 2009, then president Barack Obama signed the Family Smoking Prevention and Tobacco Control Act. This law heavily regulates tobacco advertising. American tobacco companies cannot advertise in many places including within a thousand feet of places where children gather such as playgrounds and schools. Despite these regulations, tobacco companies still manage to target young people at a very early age. According to the CDC, about seven out of ten of all middle schoolers and high school students have seen tobacco advertising. The American Academy of Pediatrics reports that even many teens who had never smoked described themselves as "highly receptive" to certain forms of tobacco advertising. Teens who felt receptive to tobacco advertising were more likely to start smoking.

Another way tobacco companies reach out to potential smokers is online. As teens spend a lot of time on home computers and iPhones, they also encounter hundreds of ads each week. Tobacco companies have jumped on the online advertising bandwagon. Clickbait—links designed to bring users to a specific web page, often with false promises—is a very common form of tobacco advertising. Much of the online tobacco advertising budget is about enticing teens to click on ads that often promise all sorts of free tobacco-related merchandise. Advertising online is also largely focused on e-cigs. Such advertising is often less regulated than other forms of advertising, allowing companies to exploit a loophole in the law and reach for websites that tend to have a higher percentage of younger visitors.

Peer Pressure

Peer pressure is another reason people start smoking. Peer pressure can play a huge role in the decision to start smoking, particularly for teens. About one-third of all American teens self-reported that they had ever tried a cigarette. Peers can vastly increase the possibility that teens will smoke at least once and continue smoking over time. Officials at the U.S. Department of Health and Human Services have found that teens who have three or more friends who are smokers are ten times more likely to smoke than teens who do not have any peers who smoke. Similar results have been found for people who are friends with those who vape. Peers who smoke can also push teens to continue to smoke even if they want to stop. Having two friends who smoke was correlated with a sixfold increase in the possibility of becoming an intermittent smoker and even more correlated with becoming a daily smoker. Parents can also play at least some role in determining if teens smoke. While boys do not appear to be influenced by parents who smoke, girls who have a mom who smokes are about a third more likely to be smokers themselves.

Educational and Self-Esteem Issues

Some people who start smoking do so because they are not aware of the actual dangers of becoming smokers. They may also disregard such health effects as something that only happens to some old people many years in the future. People who lack such awareness may also think that they can quit any time they want, so they continue to smoke. Those who do not feel connected to society and come from a disadvantaged background that discourages education may also start to smoke because it is not frowned upon in their community. A smoker may have low self-esteem. People who are overweight may choose to smoke in order to help them lose weight. Smoking can help suppress appetite in the short term. When they smoke, they feel more self-confident and more in touch with out-of-the-mainstream cultural traits. A smoker may also feel that smoking makes it easier for others to talk with them at a party or other social situations. They also eat less as smoking helps dull the appetite. Smokers may not have connections with role models who can show them why it is best to quit. Many e-cig users do not believe e-cigs are dangerous. Many parents share similar attitudes and may even vape with their teens.

Inborn Personal Traits

Smoking has been correlated with people who are more comfortable taking risks in life. Some people find it thrilling to engage in behaviors they know to be possibly dangerous. These are the same traits that may lead them to engage in other kinds of risky behavior, such as using alcohol to excess or trying other illicit substances such as heroin and cocaine. They may believe that smoking is just like behaviors that give them a sense of letting go of control such as driving too fast. The same is true for those who try e-cigs. Vaping is seen as taking a controlled risk that makes the user feel part of a different culture.

Easy Access to Cigarettes

In some communities, cigarette use is less common. A teen may only be rarely exposed to smoking and smokers. Children who see cigarettes or see an older member of the household vaping may be tempted into smoking or vaping. Where people can buy cigarettes can vary by state. In certain states such as New Jersey, people have to be at least twenty-one to buy cigarettes and other tobacco products. In other parts of the country, people can buy tobacco products as soon as they turn eighteen. These three years are often crucial. This is when people make the transition from someone who may only smoke once in a while to someone who smokes far more often. Those who can buy cigarettes legally at eighteen are far more likely to start and keep smoking than those who can't legally buy tobacco products until they turn twenty-one. In 2016, the FDA ruled it had the right to regulate the sale of e-cigs and vaping. Under this ruling, known as the Deeming Rule, vaping products cannot be sold to customers under eighteen. Some states have raised the age of legal purchase of vapor products to twenty-one. Other states are expected to follow suit. Despite this rule, teens are getting around it and finding access to vaping products on their own.

A single one of these factors can influence a person's decision to start smoking and continue smoking. More than one can make it even harder for someone to avoid smoking and harder for them to quit.

9. How does tobacco get into the body?

Many things start to happen as people smoke. The heart starts to beat faster. This brings up the heart rate and increases the blood pressure. In as little as a few seconds, the pulse starts to race. They may be briefly more alert and then drowsy. The tobacco inside their system is delivered by a complex and highly intricate biological process.

Light a cigarette, and start to smoke it, and trigger a cascade of events. A typical smoker smokes a cigarette for about five minutes. By the time the cigarette reaches the end of the flame and gets out, the typical smoker takes ten separate puffs. In the process, the smoker gets between one and two milligrams of tobacco in a few minutes. First, it enters the mouth. The mouth is a relatively delicate surface protected by a layer of saliva and other substances. Some particles of tobacco stay in the mouth and on the gums and teeth as the smoke travels through this cavity. Tobacco smoke travels further along the body into the throat as the smoker breathes. This is where the mucosal cells are found. These cells provide the lubrication the mouth needs. When the smoke continues to travel, it encounters the nasal cavity where people smell things. Smell is an integral part of what people perceive to be taste, so they may notice changes in their sense of taste and smell rather quickly. Tobacco smoke is then drawn directly into the nose from the mouth and by the heart and lungs. After the tobacco gets in the nose, it travels to the trachea or windpipe. The trachea is lined with tiny hairs that are known as cilia. They are there to keep unwanted particles out. Tobacco gets to these cells and kills them. The esophagus or food pipe is located behind the trachea and heart. It is also affected by tobacco smoke. Smoke coats the esophagus muscles as people smoke.

Right in Your Lungs and Bloodstream

While tobacco needs to travel through the mouth and nasal cavity, in order to reach the rest of the body's organs, it needs to enter the lungs. The lungs are one of the body's most complex organs. They have tubular branches that are known as bronchi. The bronchi branch into each of the two lungs separately. These get smaller and smaller. Eventually, they branch into tubes so small that they can only be seen with a microscope. These microscopic branches in the lungs cluster into tiny air sacs that are known as alveoli. This is where the breath meets the bloodstream. Oxygen and other parts of the air go from the outside and into the lungs and all the other organs of the body. Unwind them, and alveoli are actually nearly forty times the surface of the entire skin from the head to the toes. As people breathe smoke, they bring the tobacco directly from a path that leads across the mouth into the throat and into the trachea and ultimately into the lungs and then to the very center of the body.

Once tobacco smoke gets into the lungs, it's an easy path to many other organs, including the heart and brain. Tobacco gets into the blood from the lungs and binds with the blood's hemoglobin. Hemoglobin is a protein found in all red blood cells that brings oxygen to rest of the body's organs. Oxygen gives cells the energy they need to function. When tobacco gets in the bloodstream, part of the oxygen is shoved aside. Instead of the oxygen cells need, they get tobacco. Red blood cells circulate to every single organ and last about four months. Each red blood cell affected by tobacco has less room to carry oxygen because it is carrying tobacco instead. The smokers also get other chemicals in their blood as they smoke, including carbon monoxide. Carbon monoxide also gets into red blood cells and gets carried with them as the smoker inhales tobacco. From start to finish, the entire process takes only about ten seconds. It takes about eight hours for tobacco smoke to finally and fully leave the body. If the smoker chooses to smoke again, the process starts all over again.

Other Forms of Tobacco

In addition to smoking, tobacco can also get on the body and into a person's internal organs in other ways. People who harvest tobacco in the fields may not take appropriate precautions as they work. The tobacco they handle over time can be directly absorbed into the skin. If left on the skin without being scrubbed off quickly, it can also get into the rest of the body and cause problems such as the substitution of harmful chemicals for oxygen in the blood. Some people choose to use snuff or chewing tobacco. The CDC estimates that about 5 percent of all teenagers use such products on routine basis. Snuff is tobacco that is not smoked but placed against the inner part of the mouth. Just as smoke brings tobacco into other parts of the body, the same is true of using snuff. As snuff is kept in the mouth for even a few minutes, it is absorbed by the cells lining the mouth. Once absorbed, tobacco gets into the bloodstream and has many of the same effects on the body as smoking does.

10. What is secondhand smoke?

On the surface, it may seem as if the harmful effects of smoking are confined solely to the smoker. Not so. People next to the smoker are breathing in their smoke. Secondhand smoke, also known as environmental tobacco smoke or ETS, is smoke that a nonsmoker inhales involuntarily even if they never light up. They, too, will face risks over time if they are exposed to cigarette smoking. Secondhand smoke is found in many places not all of them obvious. An office worker who passes through a smoking area as they enter the building can be exposed to secondhand smoke. The waitress and bartender who serve the smoker may also be exposed to smoking. When the smoker exhales smoke, the smoke they inhale has not been purified after leaving their lungs. The smoker creates lingering trails of chemicals that can easily get absorbed into another person's organs. These chemicals continue to create a cloud of dangerous substances in the air for several feet even as the line of visible smoke seems to disappear.

Another form of secondhand smoke is known as sidestream smoke. Sidestream smoke is when the smokers light a cigar, cigarette, or pipe but do not smoke it. Instead, they may leave the lit item next to an ashtray or even set it down on the floor and not put it out. As the remaining tobacco is consumed by the flame, it releases dangerous chemicals in the immediate area. In areas where smoking is permitted, there may be dozens of smokers and large plumes of secondhand smoke in every single corner of the space.

On the surface, secondhand smoke may not seem to pose any danger. After all, nonsmokers are not lighting cigarettes and inhaling smoke. In actual practice, secondhand smoke is an extremely dangerous problem that creates risk for everyone in the immediate area. When nonsmokers wind up inhaling smoke, they are engaging in what is known as passive smoking or involuntary smoking. Many common precautions will not reduce these risks. From offering a nonsmoking dining section to opening windows or installing air filters, passive smoking is still a problem. Health professionals can determine if people have been exposed to smoking by measuring an individual's level of cotinine. Cotinine is what remains in someone's body after it has processed nicotine. One of the more insidious aspects of passive smoking is how it can affect children. Even young babies and children who have a caregiver who smokes may be at risk as they grow up. Babies with a family member who smokes are more likely to have low birth rate than babies from nonsmoking households. They are also at greater risk of problems including minor conditions such as ear infections and sore throats. Babies exposed to it also vastly increase their possibility of getting more serious medical problems such as bronchitis and pneumonia. As infants, babies living in a smoker's household are even more likely to die from a condition known as SIDS. Over time, children who grow up in a household where a smoker is present are also far more at risk for many dangerous diseases, including many types of cancers such as leukemia and lymphoma. Children who have asthma will have longer and more dangerous asthma attacks if they live with a parent who smokes.

Babies and children are not the only age group affected by passive smoking. Adults exposed to passive smoking also face enormous health risks that separate them from their peer group. About three thousand Americans get lung cancer and die each year solely because they have been exposed to passive smoking. Even if they never personally light up, adults who live with someone who smokes increase their risk of lung cancer by roughly 20 percent. Living with a smoker can also trigger heart problems in people with no other risk factors. Passive smokers experience many of the very same problems that bedevil those who actively smoke. Like active smokers, they face much greater risks of heart disease, varied types of cancers, and stroke than those who are not exposed to smoking. Just as smoking is more common among certain socioeconomic groups, the same is true of passive smoking. People who work in blue-collar occupations are more likely to be around smokers and get exposed to secondhand smoking. Ethnic minorities including African Americans are also more likely to encounter secondhand smoking. Other factors are also more likely to influence whether or not a person is exposed to passive smoking over the course of their lifetime. Renting a home or living in housing with more than one unit can increase exposure to this form of smoking. People who have a history of personal alcohol or prescription drug use are also more likely to smoke or to live with someone who does. Those with lower than average incomes are also far more likely to be exposed to secondhand smoke. Adults may also face secondhand smoke at their job. A cabbie might need to allow smokers inside to earn a daily paycheck. The cocktail waitress, daycare worker, and restaurant owner may also have no choice other than to work in such an environment.

While secondhand smoking is an ongoing problem, there is some good news. The number of people exposed to secondhand smoke has been decreasing. As fewer people smoke, fewer people around them are exposed to secondhand smoke. An increasing number of bills have been passed banning smoking in many areas. Smoking is not allowed in many places, including airplanes, hospitals, and schools. Traditional forms of smoking have also become much less socially acceptable. Many smokers no longer feel free to light up in front of others. As fewer parents smoke, babies and young children are increasingly growing up in households where they are not exposed to any form of secondhand smoke. Still, dangers persist. They are likely to continue as e-cigs and vaping also continue to be popular. Millions of people both in the United States and worldwide are exposed to secondhand smoking. A significant number of babies and children will grow up at serious risk because someone in their household smokes. Many people will suffer asthma attacks, heart attacks, and cancer as a direct result of smoking even if they do not smoke.

11. What is thirdhand smoke?

Smoking has so many hazards; it can be hard to keep track of them. One danger that is increasingly getting more attention is known as thirdhand smoke. While people have heard of the term "secondhand smoking," thirdhand smoke remains more obscure. Just like secondhand smoke, thirdhand smoke poses serious, long-term dangers that may not be immediately evident. In recent years, scientists continue to learn that any form of exposure to tobacco products is deeply detrimental. Over time, exposure to thirdhand smoke may be even more perilous than being in a room with secondhand smoke. Even short-term exposure may trigger symptoms such as coughing and shortness of breath. If you've ever walked underneath the bleachers where smokers tend to congregate and run your hands along the metal, even though there's not a puff in sight, that's thirdhand smoke. Just as people can be exposed to smoking without actually lighting up, they can also be exposed to chemicals from smoking via thirdhand smoking. The unsafe chemicals found in tobacco products linger in a room and other places such as wood park benches for years. This can happen if the room or part of the park has ever been used for smoking. The process of accumulating toxic tobacco products in a given area along all the surfaces of that room is known as thirdhand smoke. Thirdhand smoke is what happens to an area after secondhand smoke has stopped. Even when secondhand smoke is removed from spaces, it is an important concept that helps illustrate why smoking is such a truly risky endeavor. Scientists now have a better understanding of the long-term dangers smoking can pose even when the smoker is not present. Thirdhand smoke is not merely an unpleasant smell or even a temporary inconvenience. It is used to describe what happens when the dangerous chemicals found in cigarettes get on the room's indoor surfaces and fabrics and stay there.

It may seem as if smoke dissipates when it hits the air. This is not true. Tobacco smoke primarily contains gasses and what are known as particulates. Particulates are microscopic matter like soot that cling to lots of things and stay there. It may seem possible to wash and clean up the entire room or outdoor surfaces to remove such matter. However, such particles are sticky and easily cling to many surfaces and fabrics. This is why they can be hard to remove both on a daily basis and over time. Surfaces that look free from chemicals left over after smoking may not be clean at all. Particles can settle without being seen on many types of surfaces, including bedposts, a living room couch, all the kitchen countertops, and even all parts of the ceiling in the room. Another problem are gasses produced as a result of smoking. Gasses from tobacco that can be released in the atmosphere can be released into the air again. This process is known as "off gassing." The gasses from the off gassing process found in a typical puff of a cigarette can get in the lungs. They can also get in the drapes, bedding, and even clothing.

People can carry such particles with them as they travel somewhere else. In rooms where smoking is permitted, thirdhand smoke particulates can get into all the room's fabrics from the draperies to the rugs. Even a vigorous spring cleaning may not get rid of all or even most of the dangerous substances present. Thirdhand smoke can also create additional chemicals in any space by interacting with other chemicals that are already present in the atmosphere. This can lead to even more issues. The VOCs present in tobacco can interact with ozone in the air and cause yet more toxins such as formaldehyde that are known to be hazardous in large amounts. The process of cleaning surfaces can also raise dust. This dust may look harmless but is full of tobacco and other potentially cancer-causing substances. It can be very hard to fully remove the dust from the room's surfaces. A person who cleans rooms where smoking is present on a routine basis may be exposed to such chemicals as they clean each space even when the smoker is long gone. Over time, anyone who works in an area where smoking has been present at some point in time may be repeatedly exposed to serious chemicals that harm the heart, lungs, and every single organ in the body.

Because the residue from the smoke isn't easy to see, it can go unnoticed for years. Someone else may have smoked in a rental space, and you don't know about it. Chemicals from prior smoking may still be coating many surfaces in the home's rooms with an invisible chemical haze. Even if you or someone in your home does not smoke or quit smoking a long time ago, there might still have thirdhand smoke in the home. Worse still, the particulates from the smoking can form dangerous compounds. Nicotine in the leftover residue can easily react with a chemical found in most indoor spaces known as nitrous acid. Acid can cause the surfaces of the home to create noxious fumes that cause problems such as slower wound healing. In the long term, thirdhand smoke can ultimately lead to serious illnesses such as asthma and even cancer. Substances can build up over a long period of time and continue to pose a health hazard.

While it may seem as minor amounts of tobacco and other chemicals found in smoking pose no perils, it has been shown over and over again that there is never any safe level of exposure to tobacco smoke. No one should be exposed to tobacco on any occasion. Everyone has the right to an environment that does not contain noxious substances. Perhaps the worst thing about this form of smoke exposure is that people aren't even aware that they have been exposed to thirdhand smoking. Worse still, people may not take this form of smoke exposure seriously and not take proper precautions to prevent it, this despite the fact that tobacco smoke is one of the most concentrated of all toxic substances, vastly exceeding car exhaust in the sheer number of threatening chemicals found in a single cigarette.

Thirdhand smoke is a concern for all age groups. Teens should be especially aware of this issue. Thirdhand smoke poses a special danger for children and babies. Babies and young children like to put things in their mouths. Chewing on a blanket or curtain where thirdhand smoke and therefore chemicals like lead and arsenic are present can expose children and babies to substances that may have serious consequences as they grow. A child will ingest twice as much dust as any adult. They will get twice the exposure to thirdhand smoke that an adult will get. Over time, such substances can accumulate in a child's body. Worse yet, parents may not even be aware that there is a problem in the home from thirdhand smoke. Even after a parent has stopped smoking, the chemicals from smoking can still coat the walls and fabrics in their home for many months and even years. According to a paper published in the BMJ, researchers found that the homes of former smokers still had the same levels of alarming chemicals that were present when the smoker was actively smoking. When researchers examined a vacant home, they still found traces of thirdhand smoke and associated chemicals such as nicotine and tobacco even two months later. Parents who work hard to quit may still be unwittingly exposing their children and other members of their household to carcinogens. A teen's brain, unlike that of an adult, has not yet finished growing. Substances found in thirdhand smoke such as cyanide and arsenic can cause terrible problems that can prevent a teenager from reaching their full potential. Experts believe that thirdhand smoke may be even worse than secondhand smoke because secondhand smoke can largely be let out of any space via ventilation. Thirdhand smoke particulates and other dangerous substances can be trapped in many areas of the room and stay there for years before they are removed.

If you suspect the presence of thirdhand smoke in your home or any other place, it's best to deal with it immediately. If you are in a home where there's smoking or has been in the past, wash your hands completely and shower as soon as possible once you leave. Find out if someone has smoked in any part of your home. Talk to your parents. Even if they have quit, it's very easy for such thirdhand chemicals to coat many surfaces and stay there. Thirdhand smoke is a relatively recent concept that many parents do not know about. When they learn about this issue and the dangers it poses to you and your siblings, this can serve as a motivation for them to quit. A study in the journal *Pediatrics* found that parents who were educated about this matter made more of an effort to quit. They also made far more efforts to keep other areas of their homes free of smoke.

Speak with fellow students about how thirdhand smoke may be present in their homes. Keep in mind that turning on a fan or air conditioner in your home will only help spread the particulate matter and gasses, so it is not a good idea. Even if you decide to dedicate a single room solely to smoking, this may not help. Central air and central heating will circulate the smoke to other parts of the home. Airing out a room will not remove the heavy metal particles that have settled on the ceiling. The only way to get rid of any thirdhand smoke residue is to completely launder all fabric in the room and clean the entire room thoroughly, including the ceilings and windows. Acidic solutions can also get rid of thirdhand smoke from many surfaces such as marble and tile. Such acids may leave stains and may not be practical. Thirdhand smoke cannot be removed at all from wall-to-wall carpeting, so it will need to be thrown out to avoid problems. Ultimately, a smoke-free home is always the best home.

12. Are there any benefits to smoking?

The fact that smoking has many disadvantages for the smoker is well established. In the short term, smokers are at vastly increased risk of many kinds of unpleasant symptoms such as chronic cough and breathing issues. Smoking increases the heart rate and can make people feel jumpy. It can also increase blood pressure and a person's short-term risk of potentially serious cardiac events. Smoking can easily lead to coughing shortly after a smoker starts to inhale. Even a single cigarette may trigger a prolonged coughing fit. In the longer term, those who choose to smoke also face all kinds of serious health risks. Over time, smoking will vastly increase the smoker's likelihood of getting many kinds of cancers. Smokers are also at increased risk of heart attacks, strokes, and diseases that can restrict the smokers' airwaves and make it harder to breathe. Diseases such as emphysema have been directly linked to smoking. Smoking can also hurt others who live with the smoker. Children growing up with a parent who smokes face serious health risks even if they never take up smoking on their own later in life. While all this is true, many people wonder if they are any advantages to smoking. There are some benefits to smoking. When they start smoking, people often feel better, at least in the short term. This is one reason why people choose to smoke. It's also why it can be so hard to quit smoking. In general there are two types of benefits to smoking: short-term benefits and long-term benefits. While such advantages are minor and more than offset by the vast disadvantages that smokers will face as long as they continue to smoke, they are known benefits. Smoking may also help provide reduce the effects of certain chronic diseases. Many of the potential advantages of smoking come from a handful of certain chemicals that are found in smoke. Doctors are exploring ways to use the chemicals found in smoke to help provide potential benefits without the need to inhale cigarette smoke into a person's lungs.

Short-Term Effects

Smoking is a complex process that brings many chemicals into the body in a relatively short period of time. From the very first time a smoker begins to smoke, they may feel very differently. As the smoker inhales a single cigarette, they often feel an initial sense of intense and deeply pleasing relaxation. Chemicals in smoke such as nicotine immediately increase levels of chemicals already present and known to have certain, often extremely useful effects. Chemicals such as dopamine, glutamate, and endorphins are known to create effects that people enjoy. Many of these chemicals are located in primarily in the brain and can create deeply desirable states that people seek out. For example, glutamate is what is known as a neurotransmitter. A neurotransmitter is a chemical that helps make connections between cells in the body. Glutamate, for example, is known to help increase the ability to learn as well as retain what people learn. Those who smoke may initially find it easier to concentrate as they study because the chemical helps trigger increased connections between each cell. Smokers may also feel less anxious as they choose to smoke because the chemicals in the smoke help reduce their feelings of worry and fear. Paradoxically, smoking can also make people feel more awake. Smoking can offer an increase in a chemical known as adrenaline. Adrenaline, also known as epinephrine, helps make people more alert even when they might otherwise feel sleepy. This helps make smokers more aware of their surroundings no matter the time of day and gives them more energy at least on a temporary basis. The increased energy can help people respond more quickly to any complicated situation in front of them and stay alert in stressful situations such as midterms and finals. The increased temporary concentration can help the smoker do better in school and at work. In short, smokers can initially experience benefits from smoking that are very real. Such effects can lead smokers to keep smoking even when these effects wear off and other, less beneficial effects start to kick in and create unpleasant side effects.

Long-Term Benefits

In addition to some known short-term benefits, smoking may—just may—also have some important and very real long-term benefits for the smoker under certain, highly specific circumstances. It is important to keep in mind that many such effects are not entirely clear. It is also important to keep in mind that many such benefits may be attributable to other factors such as a better diet that some smokers have even as they smoke or the fact that the person chooses to exercise or simply has good genes that can help mitigate the worst effects of smoking. Just as some people can survive conditions that may easily kill others, some people who smoke may simply be lucky and better able to avoid medical conditions from smoking that will otherwise kill them, such as lung cancer. Certain medical conditions may be helped by smoking in ways that modern medical efforts cannot as yet identify or entirely explain.

Ulcerative colitis is a painful condition that can cause sores on the colon and the bowel and makes it hard for the sufferer to get through the day without embarrassing and frustrating symptoms. An October 2012 journal article in *Alimentary Pharmacology and Therapeutics* closely examined all available studies conducted on nicotine, smoking, and those suffering from this condition. They found that smoking seems to protect against the disease. Smokers were far less likely to get ulcerative colitis in the first place. They also found that smokers with ulcerative colitis experienced less pain and discomfort than those who did not smoke at all. It appears that nicotine may be able to provide help for sufferers. However, researchers also looked at another similar condition that affects the bowel. They were hoping to find that smoking might help alleviate symptoms or even ward off Crohn's disease. Researchers noted that Crohn's is similar to ulcerative colitis in that both conditions cause a person's immune system to attack the gut. In fact, they found that smoking cigarettes has been shown to exacerbate the symptoms of Crohn's disease and cause additional flare-ups. Doctors aren't sure why such similar medical problems respond so differently to smoking.

Two other diseases also illustrate the occasional paradoxes that smoking can create. Parkinson's disease and Alzheimer's disease are diseases that may strike early in life but typically strike as people age. Just like ulcerative colitis and Crohn's disease, these two diseases appear to have opposite effects when it comes to cigarette consumption. Epidemiologist Harold Kahn first noticed a connection between Parkinson's and smoking in the 1960s. He spent hours examining the records of over a quarter of million military members for over two decades. Such records are highly detailed, enabling him to have a clear record of relevant factors such as the participant's height and weight as well as any preexisting medical conditions. He found that those who smoked were actually three times less likely than those who did not to have died from Parkinson's disease. Parkinson's was less common in smokers even though they were still far more likely than nonsmokers to die from emphysema or lung cancer. Since that initial study, other studies have repeatedly born out of this connection. Parkinson's patients suffer because neurons that produce a chemical called dopamine die gradually well before they should. Researchers speculate that nicotine may decrease such degeneration. However, they do not recommend that patients suffering from Parkinson's start smoking. Alzheimer's is another degenerative brain disease. Unlike Parkinson's, smoking appears to increase the possibility that a person will get the disease. Chemicals in cigarette smoke appear to prematurely age the brain. At the same time, researchers are also exploring the possibility of using nicotine to help treat the degeneration in brain function that can develop as these diseases progress.

Obesity is another condition where paradoxes abound. People have noted that smoking cigarettes often hugely decreases a person's appetite. Many smokers are thinner than average. People will eat less because they are smoking. After they quit, many people will gain weight at least on a temporary basis. In a study published in the journal *Science* in 2011, Yale University researchers discovered that nicotine actually works by activating a specific pathway in the brain that then acts to suppress the smoker's appetite and thus leads to a decrease in weight. Now this may sound like an easy way to lose weight. At the same time, like so many claims related to this subject, further examination reveals something more troubling and more dangerous. The number of cigarettes people consume greatly varies. Some people may smoke as many as forty or even more cigarettes in a single day. Others may smoke a dozen or even far less. Those who smoke a lot are actually more likely to be obese than those who do not smoke or those who smoke more lightly. People who smoke are often of lower socioeconomic strata than those who do not smoke. They also tend to have other behaviors that can cause problems, such as a poor diet. Young people who think they can keep off the pounds by smoking also do not benefit from smoking, as a study of nearly half a million residents of the United Kingdom found in 2015.

Some other studies have found that smoking may appear to benefit people in other ways. For example, smokers may appear to survive heart attacks better than nonsmokers. At the same time, smokers also get heart attacks at a younger age than others. They are often better at surviving heart attacks because they are getting heart attacks earlier than their peers when that heart muscle is still stronger and more likely to survive the trauma of a heart attack.

It is important to look closely at all studies related to this issue. Keep in mind that many tobacco companies often fund studies on their own and may even pay respected medical researchers. Such studies are designed to illustrate that smoking actually has health benefits when it may not. Even if smoking has benefits such as the potential for weight loss, there are many ways to achieve this goal, such as eating healthier and exercising more that are far less dangerous and far healthier.

Smoking Risks

13. What are the short-term risks associated with smoking?

The long-term risks of smoking are well known. What teens may not know is that there are also many short-term risks when they choose to inhale. From the very first moment, cigarette smoke enters a person's body; it begins a series of unfortunate events. These responses affect all areas of the body from the brain to the respiratory system to the smoker's immune system and heart and digestive organs. Such risks are still being investigated, but many have been well established.

Some effects can take months to show up. At the same time, researchers at the *Chemical Research in Toxicology* found that damage to the smoker's DNA became apparent less than an hour after smoking. One of many toxic chemicals in cigarettes are polycyclic aromatic hydrocarbons or PAHs. Such chemicals have been repeatedly linked with cancer in humans. During the study, twelve volunteers agreed to smoke. They were given cigarettes with a form of PAH that can be easily identified on tests. As the smokers inhaled, it became apparent that the chemical compounds formed a toxic substance in their blood in less than an hour. This substance can enter the bloodstream and cause nearly immediate DNA damage.

Smoking also has many nearly instantaneous effects. The first effect many people notice is a feeling of relaxation. However, this feeling is deeply deceptive. As the smoker continues to inhale, even over a short period of time, they will feel a sense of anxiety as they wonder where their next smoke is coming from. The only way this feeling of desire for more tobacco and nicotine stops is when the smoker finally stops smoking for good.

Experts also believe that smoking begins to alter the brain's chemistry very early on. Studies have shown that smokers have fewer dopamine receptors in their brains. Dopamine is a chemical that has been linked with pleasurable activities such as eating. Many researchers believe that smoking destroys the amount of dopamine receptors in the brain. It is believed that smoking creating a cycle where excess dopamine is released by nicotine. Then the substance decreases the number of dopamine receptors and amount of dopamine released over time, a cycle that repeats again and again. Animal models indicate that this process begins quickly and increases over time.

When people smoke, they are also nearly instantly dragging smoke into the tiniest passages in the lungs. Tobacco smoke gets into the hairs in the lungs known as cilia and starts to paralyze them. The result? Increased mucus every time the smoker inhales. A smoker will also rapidly begin to notice more phlegm in their lungs. The best way to get it out is to cough, but coughing is now harder. They will also begin coughing even if it hurts. That is the body's response to the assault on the lungs. The smoker's heart begins to suffer. Smoking constricts the heart's vessels. Fats in your body are generally divided into fats that provide energy and those that can cause harm. From the very first, smoking brings more of the fats that can damage heart while decreasing the fats needed to power the body. Studies show that sudden death from cardiac arrest is four times more common in young men who smoke than those who don't. Even when resting and doing nothing, smoke is coursing through their blood. Thirty minutes after that first puff, nicotine has increased the resting heartbeat and made it harder to relax and concentrate.

That's not all. Other body systems also show rapid effects once people start to smoke. It's not just the heart, lungs, and brains that suffer. The rest of the body isn't much fonder of the chemicals in smoking. Smoking can quickly inflame linings in the body that keep out diseases and prevent infections. The gastrointestinal system includes several body organs such as the mouth, stomach, and intestines. Bring smoke into the stomach, and it alters the stomach's chemistry. Many smokers wind up with painful heartburn that begins shortly after they inhale. Tobacco smoke also decreases blood flow and hinders the healing of any wounds. Smoke, and you begin to increase your chances of getting painful ulcers. Smoking also gets into the oral cavity and almost immediately begins to undo daily brushing sessions by reducing the blood flow to the oral cavity. This makes it easy for harmful bacteria to settle and begin causing gum disease and discoloring the teeth. The immune system will also suffer quickly early on. This is the system that provides the first defense against extremely dangerous diseases. Smoking erodes the barriers that the body uses to keep out dangerous microbes. When people smoke, those around them tend to be far more susceptible to painful ear infections. Smoke makes it hard for the ears to prevent infectious material from getting in the ear canal. Not only might the smoker get frequent ear infections, if they smoke around your siblings, they could also have the same problems. Tobacco smoke can also easily get into sinuses. These are cavities in the skull. They're protected by the same type of hairs that line the lungs. Smoke, and you'll damage these hairs as well. Smokers may be far more vulnerable to sinusitis. Sinusitis is similar to the common cold, but it can be a lot more unpleasant. Common symptoms include headaches and ongoing facial pain. The same is true of the linings of the nasal passages and the lungs. The smoker may notice rhinitis that feels like the worst cold ever. Or worse, they may develop pneumonia and feel like an elephant is sitting on their chest.

After people start smoking, it rapidly becomes harder to get the nutrients they need each day. Smoking makes it more difficult for the body to absorb vitamins like vitamin C and vitamin E, which are necessary for good health. If the smoker has already existing medical conditions such as asthma or they are taking medications for chronic medical issues such as depression or sickle cell anemia, smoking can interfere with the body's ability to absorb these medications. Smoking can also make it harder to control type I diabetes. Are you taking hormonal birth control pills? Better use additional birth control methods if you don't want to get pregnant or get a sexually transmitted disease. Smoking will not only decrease the efficacy of the pill. It also increases the chance of serious consequences if the smoker continues to use both such as a heart attack or a stroke even if they are very young.

Some—but not all—of the effects can be reversed once the smoker quits. The seemingly short-term effects of smoking may linger and create problems long after they have left smoking behind. The best solution is to avoid smoking at all.

14. What does smoking do to the lungs?

Smoking can harm every single part of the body from the brain to the toenails. Of all the many negative effects of smoking, perhaps the most well known is that smoking damages the lungs. If people stopped smoking, lung cancer would be a very rare disease. Lung cancer is hard to treat and has a very poor prognosis. It's highly correlated with long-term smoking. Teens know that smoking increases their risk of getting lung cancer later on in life. However, many do not know what smoking or vaping actually does to their lungs. Lung cancer is very rare in young people and typically will not begin to show up until the person is well into middle age. At the same time, tobacco smoke invades every single part of the smoker's lungs. Lung damage from tobacco smoke begins the moment the smoker starts to light up. It continues as they continue to smoke. Similar issues may occur when teens use e-cigs and vape.

The lungs consist of several parts. While some people are born missing part of their lungs, most people have a right lung and a left lung. These two air-filled organs are found in your chest. People take in air via their nose and/or mouth. Air gets pulled down the windpipe or trachea. From there it travels to the bronchial tubes. At the bottom of your lungs lies the diaphragm. This is the muscle that contracts and allows people to breathe. The smallest branches of your lungs are known as alveoli or air sacs. Humans have about six hundred million of these sacs that look like bunches of grapes. They are covered in tiny veins that bring them oxygen. The lungs are covered by a membrane called the pleura. In a healthy nonsmoker, air is warmed as it gets into the lungs and then provides people with oxygen. When the smoker exhales, they are removing harmful chemicals from the body such as carbon dioxide. They are also making more difficult to smell things. This makes it harder to determine if that breakfast smells right or you need to get out the fire extinguisher because you left the pizza slice in the microwave with the tinfoil still on. Smoking interferes with this natural process. In doing so, they can easily damage every single part of their lungs. From the very first time they smoke, they may notice such effects. As people continue to smoke, they put their lungs in greater damage and create effects that can be hard if not impossible to undo.

One of the first things many smokers notice is they have more mucus. Mucus is one of the ways the body protects the lungs. This liquid is designed to trap particles before they get into the rest of the body. Smokers disrupt this natural body activity. In response, the body often produces more mucus in an effort to get rid of the toxins from the smoke. As reported in an article in the *American Journal of Respiratory and Critical Care Medicine*, researchers found that cigarette smoke will suppress a protein that acts to prevent too many mucus-producing cells from forming in the lungs. The lungs can't get rid of the mucus, so it just stays in the airwaves. This can make it harder to breathe. The smoker may develop a cough to try and expel the excess. As they do, the cough strains the lungs even further. Excessive mucus is also highly prone to infection. The lungs now have excess fluid that the smoker can't clear. Mucous picks up all sorts of microbes that will get into the rest of your systems and make you get sick.

Another way that tobacco smoke harms lungs is by literally paralyzing organs called cilia. Cilia look like little hairs under the microscope. Like mucus, they are designed to remove unwanted particles from your lungs. Tobacco smoke is poisonous for the cilia. When they stop moving, chemicals from smoke enter the lungs. Stray particles of dirt and dust can lead your lungs to clog up even more like a vacuum cleaning filter you can't empty out. For urban area smokers with lots of pollution or an area with lots of air quality issues, smoking is another way to make it harder to breathe on days when dirty air lingers on top of school and the home.

Lungs contain a protein called elastin that makes them elastic. They're designed to bend in order to allow you to inhale and exhale. Chemicals in tobacco smoke reduce the amount of elastin present. Over time, they make it harder for your lungs to move. If you could take your lungs and unfold them, they'd take up about fifty to seventy-five meters or about seven hundred square feet. That's enough to cover a tennis court. Smokers destroy parts of these tissues making the lungs far less efficient. To get enough oxygen into the lungs, people need all this space. They also need this space to remove all the gasses like carbon dioxide. Over time, smoking reduces the ability to move the lungs and destroy parts of it such as the cilia. Smoking also damages those tiny air sacs. These sacs now hold less air and also make it harder to breathe.

Any kind of smoking puts the smoker at risk for several kinds of lung diseases. According to the Mayo Clinic, over two hundred thousand cases of lung cancer are diagnosed annually. Estimates indicate that about 90 percent of all cases of lung cancer are caused by smoking. Men are particularly at risk as they are about 23 percent more likely to develop lung cancer if they smoke. Women who smoke are about thirteen times more likely to get lung cancer. Another type of lung disease linked with smoking is chronic obstructive pulmonary disease or COPD. COPD is one of the nation's leading causes of death. This disease is divided into two types. Chronic bronchitis is an inflammation of the bronchial tubes. Symptoms include chest pain, a painful cough, and wheezing. Emphysema is another form of COPD. Emphysema is a chronic medical condition that can worsen over time and make it hard for people to breathe at all unless they're tethered to an oxygen machine. Smokers are also at increased risk for pneumonia, an infection of the lungs. Smokers are ten times more likely to get COPD than those who've never smoked.

If you want to protect your lungs, it's best to avoid smoking altogether. The sooner you quit, the more opportunity you give your lungs to heal.

15. What does smoking do to the heart?

The heart is the single most important organ in the body. As the body's pump, it ensures that your body stays alive. The heart removes the body's carbon dioxide and ensures that blood gets to other organs. Humans cannot survive without a heart. The heart is very vulnerable to tobacco smoke. Teens are aware that smoking can harm their lungs. What they may not know is that smoking can also harm their heart and their entire circulatory system just as much if not more than the lungs.

The cardiovascular system consists of the heart, vessels that carry blood, and the blood that flows through them. The heart is in the middle of the chest. It's behind and a little bit to the left of the breastbone or sternum and covered in a delicate sac known as the pericardium. The pericardium connects the heart with other parts of the body including the spinal column. This vitally important organ is about the size of a fist. Depending on the person's age and sex, a standard heart weighs between 7 and 15 ounces, or between 200 and 425 grams. Look inside the organ, and there are four chambers. Each chamber is divided into a left side and a right side. The upper two chambers are known as the atria. The bottom two chambers are the heart's ventricles. The heart has four main blood vessels. These are the vena cava, pulmonary artery, pulmonary vein, and the aorta. Smokers interfere with the heart's ability to pump blood and remove wastes.

Experts estimate that about 20 percent of all deaths from heart disease can be directly attributed to smoking. Smokers increase the heart rate making the organ work harder to pump blood. Tobacco and other chemicals in the smoke make all four of the heart's major arteries get much narrower. This can cause an irregular heart rhythm and trigger a fatal heart attack. Tobacco smoke also increases blood pressure, leading an increased possibility of a stroke. Chemicals in the smoke get into the heart's arteries and lead to a buildup of a substance known as plaque. Plaque impedes the blood flow to and from the heart and can lead to several kinds of serious heart conditions. Smoking increases levels of a substance called cholesterol, as well as a type of dangerous blood fat called triglycerides. Substances can stick to the walls of the arteries. Smoking also decreases a type of substance called high-density lipoproteins (HDL). This is what keeps artery walls in good shape. Smoking lowers levels of fibrinogen. Fibrinogen helps the body avoid dangerous blood clots that can also increase the risk of a heart attack or stroke.

Two substances in cigarette smoke are responsible for much of the damage done by smoking. Nicotine creates what is known as a "fight or flight" reaction. This is when people feel primed for action. In response, the body releases fat into your bloodstream. Stored fats stick to the walls of the heart's arteries and stay there. It makes the body produce excessive adrenaline, which can lead to problems such as elevated blood pressure. Another substance found in tobacco smoke is carbon monoxide. Carbon monoxide binds to the hemoglobin in blood. This molecule carries the blood's oxygen supply. As it does, it decreases the amount of oxygen delivered to cells. When there's an oxygen deficit, the heart has to work harder. As a result, over time it may get dangerously enlarged. Lack of oxygen can cause the heart to beat faster, thus aging it even more.

Smoking has also been implicated in many kinds of heart disease. Smoke reduces the amount of oxygen getting in the blood. Nicotine in smoking reduces the elasticity of the heart's blood vessels making it harder for the vessels to contract as the heart pumps. Nicotine can make it more likely that these vessels will weaken over time. As they do, smokers develop a disease known as arteriosclerosis when arteries hardened. Hardened arteries make it harder to get blood to the body's organs. Over time, it can damage the heart and can lead to further damage to other parts of the body such as the kidneys or brain. Smokers double their risk of a heart attack.

They also vastly increase the risk of coronary heart disease and strokes. Strokes are the fifth leading cause of death in the United States. Strokes happen when an artery leading to the brain is blocked off. Cells in the brain can die rapidly. Smoking triples the risk of a stroke. Smokers are also three times more likely to die after what is known as a sudden cardiac death. Sudden cardiac death is not what people think about when they hear the term "heart attack." It's when the heart's electrical system begins misfiring. The sufferer's heart starts to beat dangerously fast and fails to pump blood to the rest of the body. It's a medical emergency. Without rapid treatment, the sufferer may die. Unlike heart attacks, sudden cardiac death, while rare in children, may strike people in their thirties and forties. Those who smoke are also at fivefold risk of getting peripheral artery disease. This condition means that blood flow is reduced in the arteries that lead to their limbs. Smokers may have pain when they walk or find it hard to use their hands to do things such as typing or even getting dressed.

It's not only the heart that's at risk from smoking. Others who inhale smoke may also develop heart disease because of tobacco smoke. An article published in the medical journal *Circulation* called "The Cardiovascular Risk in Young Finns Study" followed about twenty-five hundred children for over a quarter of a century. When the study first began, researchers took the level of nicotine in the participants' blood. They also closely questioned all the parents about each child's level of exposure to cigarette smoke. Over two decades later, they examined the level of plaque in the children's arteries. They were startled to find that children living in a household where at least one parent smoked were 70 percent more likely to develop plaque than those who lived in a smoke-free home.

Vaping and the use of e-cigs have also been tied to an increased risk of stroke and heart disease. Officials examined the 2016 Behavioral Risk Factor Surveillance System. This is a survey that is part of the U.S. Centers for Disease Control and Prevention (CDC). Researchers looked at over sixty-six thousand people who said they had vaped. They were compared with those who had never used such methods. They found users had a 71 percent greater risk of stroke, 59 percent greater risk of heart attack, and a 40 percent increased risk of heart disease compared to those who did not use e-cigs. The study was published in the October 2018 issue of the *American Journal of Preventive Medicine*.

When you quit smoking and use e-cigs, you're reducing your risks of a heart attack and other cardiac complications. You're also helping others around you keep their hearts healthy.

16. What does smoking do to the brain?

In many ways, the brain is who we are. This is where emotions, thoughts, perceptions of the world, and personality exist. In one sense, the brain is you, and the rest of your body merely houses a few appendages. Get a heart transplant, a new kidney, or lungs from someone else, and you'll still be you. Remove your brain, and that's the end of your existence as a person. Just as smoking and vaping can hurt so many other parts of the body from your eyes to the heart and pancreas, smoking can harm the brain as well.

The brain is divided into the cerebrum, the cerebellum, and the brain stem. The cerebrum is the largest section of the brain. It's composed of right and left hemispheres. The cerebrum is where all senses get processed. This is the part of your brain that sees a sunset, hears a choir, smells dinner, feels a kitten, and knows your fingers are knitting a new hat for your nephew's birthday. This is also the part of your brain that makes judgments like determining if you should cross the street. Here's where you respond to stress and feel love when your boyfriend sends you a romantic text. The cerebellum is responsible for coordinating your muscle movements. It keeps your posture upright and makes sure you don't topple over as you move. The brain stem is the smallest part of your brain and connects the brain to the spinal column. If you've ever wondered why you usually don't have to think about breathing or maintaining your heartbeat, the brain stem is the part of your body that does that for you. The human brain is further divided into four lobes: the frontal lobe, parietal lobe, occipital lobe, and temporal lobe. These lobes perform specific functions including speech, self-awareness, memory, and your ability to concentrate. Smoking can harm all sections of the brain. It can interfere with heartbeat, memory, and spatial perception.

Over time, researchers have found that smoking impairs the brain in dozens of ways. A study in the journal *Molecular Psychiatry* actually found that cigarettes can literally shrink the brain. Over time, people who smoke have thinner than average cortexes. In a very real sense, if this part of the brain is broken, the whole brain is broken. The only way to bring back the cortex to a normal size is to stop smoking and keep stop smoking. Even then, it can take as long as a decade for the cortex to be comparable in size to the cortexes of nonsmokers. Another study examined the brains of teens. The brains of teens continue to develop for years even after you leave high school. Right now, your brain is a work in progress. Substances in tobacco smoke can hamper brain development. Researchers at the Semel Institute for Neuroscience and Human Behavior at University of California, Los Angeles, looked at the brains of twenty-five teen smokers and twenty-five teen nonsmokers. Using a measure called the Heaviness of Smoking Index, they measured the levels of nicotine dependence in all of their smoking subjects. They found that the more the teens smoked, the less activity they showed in the prefrontal cortex. The prefrontal cortex is a particularly important area of the brain for adolescents. This is the part of the brain that helps make important decisions. As such, teens rely on it heavily for the rest of their lives. Studies show that this part of the brain does not finish growing until people are about twenty-five. This is why teens tend to make different decisions than adults. People use this part of the brain to do things such as decide on a career, determine if it makes sense to run that red light, or wait for it to change and help them figure out how to respond to difficult situations and exert impulse control. Smoking ultimately makes it harder for teens to access the brain power they need to make good life choices such as paying attention in English class and not driving over the speed limit. Teens who choose to smoke as adolescents not only may impair their decision-making processes but also can create deficits that will continue as they grow up. Nicotine directly acts on the areas of the brain responsible for cognitive and emotional maturation. Teen smokers are also at increased risk of psychiatric disorders later on in life. Teens' brains are more plastic than the brains of adults. Neuroscientists have demonstrated that this is a time in life when new synaptic connections between brain cells and new firing patterns are being made. Learning at this time of your life can be much easier now than it will be when you get older. Exposure to nicotine reduces the ability to make such synaptic connections and ultimately reduces long-term ability to learn new things.

Smoking has also been heavily implicated in many diseases of the brain. A cerebral aneurysm is when the brain's blood vessels weaken. Cerebral aneurysms are very dangerous, often leading to strokes and deaths. Researchers at the Pennsylvania State University College of Medicine have suggested that smoking can not only cause such aneurysms to form but also increase the likelihood they'll rupture with devastating consequences. Smokers also face vastly increased chances of strokes, Alzheimer's disease, and dementia. Strokes happen when blood supply is cut off to the brain. A stroke can be fatal or can leave people unable to speak or move one side of their body. Alzheimer's disease and dementia are diseases of the brain that destroy memories, make it hard for people to do things such as driving, and may even make it impossible for sufferers to recognize their closest relatives. People with Alzheimer's disease will ultimately die sooner than their peers. Scientists believe that roughly 14 percent of all cases of Alzheimer's disease are directly attributable to smoking. People don't need to smoke directly to have brains that are damaged by smoking. A study in the *Archives of General Psychiatry* found that nicotine can get into the brains of a significant percentage of nonsmokers merely by being in a car with a smoker for an hour. Tobacco smoke can hurt the brain. Smokers damage their very ability to learn and make good choices in adolescence. Over time, smoking harms the structure of the brain. Smoking makes it more likely that people will suffer diseases of the brain. As it does, it makes it more likely that they'll ultimately destroy the part of themselves that make them who they are.

Vaping also poses special dangers for the brain. A study in the journal *Environmental Health Perspectives* examined fifty-six e-cigarette devices from people who vape. They also examined the "refilling dispenser, aerosol, and remaining e-liquid in the tank." A close examination revealed that the e-cig devices produced vapors that presented huge risks for users. About half of the devices produced lead well in excess of amounts known to be safe. Lead is especially injurious to babies, teens, and young children. As the authors point out, "Lead is a known neurotoxicant, which means that the health effects are on the brain directly, and the developing brains of younger adults—or the kids—have the highest susceptibility." Even more startling, a full 40 percent of the samples from vaping contained excess levels of the mineral manganese. Manganese is known to potentially trigger a condition called manganism. This condition resembles Parkinson's disease in the way that it can cause deterioration of brain cells. Vapers not only put themselves at risk from such conditions. They also put others in the room with them at risk as the vapors can get on the surfaces in the rooms where people vape.

17. Can smoking cause lung cancer?

Like the heart, the lungs power the body. Lungs are light, air-filled sacs. Unlike other organs, place them in water and they'll float. Over the course of a lifetime, people breathe in and out over half a million times. Many diseases interfere with this process. One of the most devastating and deadly is lung cancer. According to the American Cancer Society, lung cancer is the second-most common cancer for both men and women. About 14 percent of all new cases of cancer are lung cancer. In the United States alone, each year roughly a quarter of million people will be diagnosed with lung cancer. About a hundred and fifty thousand people die from it annually. A number of factors have been linked with the risk of getting lung cancer. People who are exposed to a dangerous, colorless gas called radon as well as those who have been exposed to radiation treatment for cancer in the past are all at risk. People who have had lung cancer in the past may develop a new lung cancer. Those who have relatives who've had lung cancer are also known to be at risk of developing themselves.

While these factors can contribute to cases, by far the number one cause of lung cancer is smoking. Experts state that lung cancer would be a very rare disease if no one smoked at all. Lung cancer typically exhibits few, if any, symptoms in the early stages. By the time symptoms show up, in most cases it's too late for a cure. Officials at the CDC estimate that smoking cigarettes is responsible for about 80 to 90 percent of all cases of lung cancer. Those who smoke are between 15 and 30 percent more likely to get lung cancer or to die from the disease than nonsmokers. People who choose to use pipes and other forms of tobacco products also face increased risks of getting lung cancer and dying from it. Even when people quit, they still have an elevated risk of getting lung cancer over time. Those who smoke the longest and smoke the most tobacco products are the most at risk. Even smoking just a few cigarettes or using a small bit of tobacco on a weekly basis can still vastly elevate a person's risk of lung cancer when compared to those who have never smoked at all. Secondhand smoke can also cause lung cancer. Breathing in any form of tobacco, whether from a lit cigarette, cigar, or pipe, can hurt all those around the smoker. According to the CDC, each year over seven thousand people who have never smoked die from lung cancer solely because others around them have done so. Living with a smoker means that the nonsmoker increases someone's personal chance of getting lung cancer by about 20 to 30 percent in the long run.

That smoking causes lung cancer is well known. What is also well known is very much exactly how smoking causes this form of cancer. The process of causing lung cancer begins when the chemicals in tobacco get into the lungs and damage the cells that line your lungs. There are over seven thousand chemicals in tobacco smoke. Of these, many such as tar, nickel, arsenic, and formaldehyde are known to cause cancer in the doses that smokers inhale or bring into their internal organs. The chemicals found in tobacco also work in combination to disrupt important bodily processes. For example, dangerous levels of chromium make other poisons already found in cigars, cigarettes, and many other tobacco products such as benzo[a]pyrene not only enter the body more easily but also more likely to stick more strongly to the body's DNA. These chemicals disrupt the genes that are responsible for both healthy cell growth and healthy cell division. They literally disrupt the genes in the DNA that check cell growth. When a healthy cell is damaged, it will divide in order to repair that damage. After the cell is healthy again, the cell will stop dividing. However, cancer cells continue to divide even when damage is present in the cells. Once genes can no longer control the growth of cell division, it's easy for cells to begin growing out of control and form cancerous masses. Studies have found that most people will get one mutated cell in their body for every fifty cigarettes they smoke. Over time, as they continue to smoke, this process of cell division and cell damage from such mutations can lead to a huge increase in the person's chances of cancerous cells and lung cancer. In many instances, the body can head cancer cells off at the pass and remove them. Smoking disrupts the process of removing such cells and makes it more likely that they will stick around and form tumors.

Interfering with healthy cell growth is bad enough. The damage from cigarettes and other tobacco products doesn't stop there. Chemicals in tobacco products also cause inflammation. Inflammation is a crucial and necessary body process by itself. Substances such as hormones and white blood cells use this process to help heal wounds. However, when the body constantly experiences such problems, over time inflammation continues and the process of healing becomes less efficient. Researchers at the University of Alabama at Birmingham found that cigarette smoke shuts off a key enzyme in the airways. This enzyme is known to regulate the body's ability to respond to inflammation. Chronic inflammation in the lungs makes it easier for cancer to grow. It also makes it easier for lung cancers to grow fast and begin to spread to other parts of the body. Lung cancer can take decades to show up. Preliminary evidence indicates that e-cigs are just as harmful to the lungs as other forms of smoking. A study by the Center for Tobacco Control Research and Education at the University of California, San Francisco, found that e-cigs disrupt the chemical balance of the lungs in the same way that smoking standard cigarettes does. E-cigs also produce chemicals called acetals. These chemicals greatly irritate the lungs and kill the lungs' cells.

Some people can smoke for years and even decades and yet never get lung cancer. However, over time, many people who smoke are not as lucky. They will get lung cancer, and they die from it. Of all the forms of cancer that have been studied, lung cancer is perhaps the one that is easiest to avoid.

18. Is smoking linked to any other kinds of cancer?

Cancer is a dangerous and often deadly group of related diseases. Cancer can strike any organ in the body, from the spine to the heart, pancreas, and brain. Essentially cancer is a disease of uncontrolled growth. As cells grow, they turn into cells that perform necessary functions such as breathing, fighting off invading viruses, and digesting food. Cells grow by dividing. A typical cell will divide about fifty times before it dies. When cells die, other healthier cells replace them. In turn, the no longer healthy cells are discarded. What happens as a result of a cancer is that damaged cells do not die off. Instead, they continue to divide. People can get cancerous tumors. Tumors can reduce the blood supply to their vital organs and spread the damaged cells to other parts of the body. A liver tumor may spread to the brain and stomach. Tumors can make it hard to breathe, fight off infectious diseases, and can interfere with a person's ability to move, swallow food, or see. Officials at the American Cancer Society state that cancer is the nation's second-most common cause of death. Over the course of a lifetime, about 40 percent of all Americans will get some form of cancer. Scientists believe there are more than two hundred types of cancers. Some of the most common types of cancers are skin cancer, breast cancer, leukemia, and prostate cancer. Smoking has been repeatedly shown to trigger many types of cancers. Smoking causes cancers by putting known carcinogens in the body. With each puff, toxins come in contact with a smoker's cells. Over time, such exposure triggers cell damage. Smoking damages the body's DNA and the body's ability to remove damaged cells. Damaged cells can easily multiply over time. As they do, they can create cancerous tumors that have been formed because of the chemicals in tobacco smoke and the nicotine found in e-cigs.

As explored in the previous question, smoking has been shown to cause lung cancer. If people did not smoke, lung cancer would not be the second-most common kind of cancer for both men and women. Lung cancer is what many teens think about when they think about smoking and cancer. While smoking is responsible for most cases of lung cancer, it's also heavily related to the person's chances of getting other types of cancers. Scientists who study this issue believe that smoking can cause many types of cancers, including blood cancer, bladder cancer, cervical cancer, colorectal cancer, esophageal cancer, kidney cancer, liver cancer, mouth cancer, and cancers of the pancreas, stomach, and throat. People don't need to smoke tobacco to get cancer from using tobacco or vaping. Place it in the mouth, and the user upped their chances of getting mouth cancers, cancer of the throat, and other types of soft tissue cancer. Vape or use e-cigs, and get a similar level of exposure. About one in three cases of cancer are directly linked to smoking and therefore preventable. One out of every five cancer deaths are also directly linked to smoking and also completely preventable. Health officials believe that smoking is responsible for about 20 percent of all cases of stomach cancer, 77 percent of all cases of larynx cancers, and more than half of all cases of oral cavity, pharynx, and esophageal cancers. Smokers have a fivefold risk of developing bladder cancer over those who do not smoke. Smokers are also two to three times more likely to get pancreatic cancer, a cancer that is hard to find and even harder to treat. Eighty-five percent of all cases of head and neck cancers are linked to smoking. Health officials also believe that smoking is responsible for 12 percent of colorectal cancer and 25 percent of all cases of AML or acute myelogenous leukemia. Health officials have discovered that girls who smoke as teens may be more likely to develop premenopausal breast cancer. Women who smoke for decades have been shown to be twice as likely to get ovarian cancer as those who did not. A study in the *Archives of Dermatology* by researchers at the University of Nottingham in England found that smokers have a more than 50 percent increase compared to nonsmokers for a serious form of skin cancer called squamous cell carcinoma.

Smoking not only increases a person's chances of getting cancer. It also increases the chances that the methods used to fight cancer such as radiation and chemotherapy will be less effective. Treatment for cancer, while ultimately upping long-term survival rates in many cases, may have serious side effects that make such treatment hard and uncomfortable for many patients. Problems such as fatigue, nausea, sleep disruptions, memory problems, and cognitive impairments are all commonly seen in patients being treated for cancer. Studies have repeatedly found that smokers undergoing treatment for smoking-related cancers will suffer from such treatment side effects more often. They've also found that such side effects tend to be of longer duration and may even last long after the treatment is complete. This leads some cancer patients to quit the very chemotherapy that might have saved their lives. Researchers have also found that even if the treatment works initially, smoking can increase the chances of a second bout of cancer over time. Nicotine, found in e-cigs as well as standard cigarettes, is believed to increase blood flow to cancerous tumors. This can make it easier for cancer to metastasize to the rest of the body and ultimately kill people. Smoking also interferes with the body's ability to heal after surgery to remove a cancerous tumor. When cancer sufferers quit, they decrease the treatment's risk of serious side effects and make it more likely that the treatment will beat back their tumors. They also increase their overall long-term survival rates and decrease the chances the cancer will come back.

19. What other diseases and conditions are linked to smoking?

Smoking has been linked to many illnesses, both chronic and acute. Inhale smoke, and you're putting chemicals in your body that can and will cause harm. Over time they will compromise your ability to walk, hear, breath, taste, and even think. Get pregnant, and smoking will harm also the baby and cause chaos in the womb the moment you take that first drag.

Acid Reflux

Acid reflux is when the acid already in the stomach leaks upward into the esophagus. Sometimes it has no symptoms. Other times, sufferers get painful heartburn that can keep them up all night and into the morning. Nicotine relaxes the ring of muscle that leads from the esophagus into the stomach. It may also cause the mouth to make less saliva, leading to worse heartburn. If you'd like to enjoy that pizza and ice cream without pain, avoid the cigarette smoke.

Age-Related Macular Degeneration, Cataracts, Conjunctivitis, and Glaucoma

The delicate eyes are particularly sensitive to smoking. Cataracts and glaucoma are some of the most common eye diseases. Over time, pressure can build and destroy vision from glaucoma. Cataracts are when part of the eye clouds over. Age-related macular degeneration (AMD) makes it harder to see as you get older. Smoking doubles the risk of getting a cataract and increases a person's chances of getting AMD and glaucoma. Smoke around a little sister or brother? You've increased their chances of getting painful pink eye.

Asthma

Asthma is one the nation's most common chronic medical conditions. Roughly twenty-five million Americans or one in twelve suffer from asthma. Asthma happens when the airways in the lungs narrow and swell. The respiratory system produces extra mucus. This can impede your breathing and make it hard to catch your breath. Asthma sufferers are particularly in danger from smoking as their airways are already overreactive to outside elements. Smoking makes it much harder to control asthma and harder to prevent asthma attacks. A study in the journal *Chest* found "secondhand exposure to vaping [to] raise the chances of asthma attacks in adolescents with the respiratory condition. Middle school and high school students with asthma were 27 percent more likely to have suffered an asthma attack if they'd been exposed to vapor from someone else's e-cigarette use, the researchers found."

Cleft Palate

A cleft palate is a disfiguring and painful birth defect. According to the CDC, mothers who smoke early in pregnancy are about 6 percent more likely to give birth to babies with this defect.

Crohn's Disease

Crohn's disease is an inflammation of the digestive system. Over time, it can cause all kinds of symptoms including bleeding, abdominal cramps, and fever. Those who smoke are more likely to develop Crohn's disease. They are also more likely to develop more severe symptoms than those who don't smoke.

Dementia

Dementia is a degenerative brain disease. People with dementia have trouble remembering basic facts about their own lives. As the disease gets worse and worse, they may not be able to recognize the faces of their loved ones. Continue smoking, and over time you'll increase your chances of spending your old age forgetting who you are.

Diabetes

Diabetes is a serious disease that happens when the pancreas malfunctions. Over time, diabetes can destroy just about every organ. Diabetes is generally divided into two types. Type I is typically found in children and young adults. Type II diabetes is usually found in older adults. Smoking can harm people with type I diabetes by making treatment less effective. Studies have found that smoking is linked to dangerous low glucose levels that can make people with type I diabetes find it hard to function. Smoking can actually trigger type II diabetes. Those who smoke are about thirty to forty times more likely to get type II diabetes than nonsmokers. The greater number of cigarettes smoked, the higher the risk of type II diabetes. Smoking can also make it harder to control diabetes and make serious side effects such as blindness and amputation even more likely. The nicotine found in e-cigs can also contribute to additional problems for those with either type of diabetes.

Ectopic Pregnancy

An ectopic pregnancy is when a fertilized egg implants somewhere outside of the uterus. Ectopic pregnancies are a medical emergency. Without proper treatment, women are at risk from conditions ranging from the loss of a fallopian tube to hemorrhages and even death. Smokers quadruple their risk of an ectopic pregnancy.

Hearing Loss

The ears tell you a lot about the world. Tobacco smoke contains substances that are known to be ototoxic or cause hearing loss. A study in the *Journal of the American Medical Association* found that smokers were 70 percent more likely to have at least some form of hearing loss than those who did not smoke. Smoke a lot, and you'll damage the ears even more. Hang out with smokers, and, even if you don't smoke, you'll also risk hearing loss. Nicotine like that found in vaping restricts blood flow to the ears. Research has shown that hearing isn't fully developed until late adolescence. Vaping now can affect the ability to hear for the rest of the vaper's life.

Infertility

Smoking can affect the chances of conceiving a baby. Women who are smokers typically take longer to get pregnant. Smoking can damage a man's sperm count. It can also make sperm less likely to fertilize an egg. Women who smoke may lose their store of healthy eggs more quickly than those who don't. Smoking can also trigger a condition known as premature ovarian failure in a woman's daughter, making it more likely she'll be in menopause much earlier than her peers. A study at the University College London found that "men who smoke electronic cigarettes have less potent and a lower quantity of sperm than the average male, making it more difficult for them to father a child." This is true even for males who used e-cigs that don't contain nicotine. The flavorings can also harm sperm potency and production.

Lupus

Lupus is a chronic autoimmune disease. Over time, sufferers may have swollen joints, fatigue, hair loss, skin rashes, and painful breathing. Fifteen thousand Americans will get a lupus diagnosis each year. According to the Lupus Foundation of America, "It's clear that smoking complicates and accelerates the ill effects of lupus." Smoking can make treatment less effective and worsen side effects.

Osteoporosis

As people get older, their bones can get weaker. Osteoporosis is the medical term for this condition. Roughly forty-four million people have osteoporosis in the United States. Women live longer and have less bone mass than men, so they are more vulnerable. Smokers typically experience more bone loss over a quicker period of time in comparison with nonsmokers. Smokers are also more at risk from fractures and will heal more slowly when they get them than nonsmokers.

Premature Baldness and Gray Hair

Your hair is your crowning glory. If you'd like to keep it, you're better off not smoking. Smoking damages hair follicles and prevents them from growing back. Women who smoke may also lose their hair and see their remaining curls go gray at an early age. The nicotine found in e-cigs has the same effect.

Psoriasis

When skin cells form itchy patches, that's psoriasis. Psoriasis can consist of a few minor areas or cover large parts of the skin. It can also flare up and then go into remission. Studies indicate smoking doubles the risk of psoriasis. Smokers also experience higher rates of flair-ups and have fewer remissions than nonsmokers. Studies have also indicated that heavy smokers have twice the risk of severe cases when compared to those who have never smoked.

Rheumatoid Arthritis

Rheumatoid arthritis is an autoimmune disease. The body's own immune system attacks the lining of the joints. This can cause pain and make it hard for people to move. Smokers and vapers have an increased risk of developing rheumatoid arthritis as well as an increased risk of more severe symptoms. Smokers may also have a reduced chance of responding to the medications used to treat it.

20. What role do genetics play in the likelihood that negative health effects will result from smoking?

Genes are the building blocks of all life. They perform many roles. Nearly every nucleus in every cell of your body contains genes. Genes build bones, let you move around with ease, digest your food, and make sure the lungs take in air and the heart continues to beat at a steady pace. Everyone gets half their genes from one parent and half the genes from another. Everyone also has a unique combination of genes. When people are conceived, they get the basic blueprints. As they grow, genes may be influenced in certain ways. Even if a person has a specific gene, this may not mean they will exhibit a certain trait as genes can be modified by certain factors. For example, if someone has the genes to be taller than average, this may not mean they will become tall. During the winter of 1944–1945, as World War II continued, the German army blockaded many provinces in the northern Netherlands. As a result, there was a severe food shortage in the country. Thousands of people died from starvation. The Netherlands is a highly developed country with typically low infant mortality rates and high individual income levels. As such, residents of the Netherlands are typically healthy and often taller than other nationals. Such was not the case, however, for those babies born during this period. The Dutch Famine Birth Cohort Study under the auspices of the Clinical Epidemiology and Biostatistics, Gynecology and Obstetrics and Internal Medicine of the Academic Medical Centre in Amsterdam, along with the MRC Environmental Epidemiology Unit of the University of Southampton in Britain, discovered many disturbing facts about children born during this time. In general, babies born to mothers who were part of the starved regions were shorter and had much greater chances of chronic health problems. In a sense, while genes are possibilities and probabilities, they are not necessarily destiny.

Smokers face an increased risk of getting heart attacks and strokes. They are more likely to get many types of cancers, including lung cancer and breast cancer as well as certain types of skin cancers. Those who smoke are also at risk from conditions such as hearing loss, vision problems, fertility issues, and chronic coughs. Scientists once thought that genes were unalterable and stayed static for a person's entire life. Today, researchers know genes can be changed even after a person is conceived and born. When people smoke, they can actually alter their own genetic makeup. In a study in Sweden by the Uppsala University and Uppsala Clinical Research Center, researchers were able to demonstrate that smoking can change your genes. When people smoke, genes that are designed to protect the human body from conditions such as lung cancer and heart attacks are disabled.

Another study at the Los Alamos National Laboratory examined the kind of damage that smoking can do to a person's DNA and their genes. People who have been smoking a pack a day for years are literally at risk from all kinds of changes to the body's chemistry and the genes they've inherited. A mutation is a change in the very structure of a gene. Mutations can also be inherited by the person's offspring. The study found that smoking can lead to about a hundred and fifty mutations in the lungs alone. Possible gene damage does not end there. Smoke a single pack of cigarettes every day for a year. Doing so produces nearly a hundred mutations in each cell of the larynx. It creates 23 mutations in each cell of the mouth, 18 mutations in the bladder, and 6 in each cell in the liver. Scientists know that mutations in the cell are what cause cells to become cancerous. Substances in smoking break down the body's defense against cell changes and uncontrolled growth. The result is that smokers are at greatly increased risk for many kinds of cancers largely because they have smoked and continue to smoke. Smoking essentially creates scars in DNA that can be measured over time. Quit smoking, and some of these scars may fade and even disappear. However, a study in the American Heart Association journal *Circulation: Cardiovascular Genetics* looked at sixteen thousand people and their genes. Blood samples found that smokers who quit had healed some of the damage to their DNA by about five years after they'd stopped smoking. At the same time, a significant number of genes remained changed, indicating that the person would be susceptible to many negative health effects over time, including certain cancers, strokes, and COPD. Those who continued to smoke showed alterations in over seven thousand genes or a full third of all human genes.

It's not just the smoker's DNA that can get negatively altered as they continue to smoke. Researchers at the University of California, San Francisco, found that smokers can also alter the genes of their fetuses. Smoking apparently leads to deletions in the child's genetic code. When a child has parts of the genes that are involved in their immune cell development, that child may be more vulnerable to the most common type of childhood cancer. Acute lymphoblastic leukemia or ALL strikes over three thousand American children and teens each year. Researchers found that most children with ALL had tumors with genetic deletions. The most serious genetic damage was found in mothers who smoked. Fathers who smoke also had a higher risk of offspring with such deletions.

Smoking can change just about all the cells in the body in a negative way. It can also cause problems for the person's children. Smoking and e-cigs can harm that child's genes if the person smokes during pregnancy or after the baby is born.

21. Will smoking hurt me and the baby if I get pregnant?

Roughly 14 percent of American women are smokers. When women smoke, they aren't just risking their own health. They're also risking the health of their future children. Many women don't know they're pregnant for a long time. They may have been pregnant for several weeks before they get a blood test or begin to suspect they're going to have a baby. Smoking can harm a fetus even before the woman conceives and as the pregnancy continues. Many chemicals found in tobacco smoke are not only dangerous in the womb but may also cause lasting problems as a child grows into adulthood. When you smoke, your baby inhales the same dangerous chemicals that you do. Just as smoking can cause problems with internal organs, it can also do the same to the body's organs during the vulnerable time when they are first being formed.

The damage that smoking does begins even before the woman gets pregnant. A study in the University of the Saarland, Homburg/Saar, Germany, found that smoking creates sperm that has too little of a certain protein called protamine 2. Men who smoke can have problems with sperm that are unable to fertilize eggs. Women who smoke can have trouble getting pregnant. Smoking can interfere with many female reproductive organs. Smoking can also cause an increased risk of ectopic pregnancy and thus issues with blocked and damaged fallopian tubes. If a woman does get pregnant, if she smokes, she's at greater risk of a miscarriage during all three trimesters.

One of the biggest problems that smoking can cause is what is known as low birth weight. Smoking has been linked to an increase in preterm labor. Preterm labor is when a woman gives birth before thirty-seven weeks gestation. Premature labor carries many risks for the babies. It can cause a mom to give birth before the baby has organs that are fully developed and has a layer of fat to help them regulate their temperature. Babies need to gain weight in the womb. A baby born weighing under five pounds can have many long-lasting health issues. Studies have shown that smoking is linked to giving birth to a baby with low birth weight. Low birth weight is associated with complications such as difficulties feeding properly, breathing complications, and an increased risk of infections. Babies who are born with low birth weight may suffer from chronic issues as they grow older including developmental delays, heart issues, and problems with their hearing and sight. Low birth weight also puts babies at risk from dying before they're a year old. Smoking has also been linked to a condition called SIDS. SIDS is short for sudden infant death syndrome. Chemicals in cigarette smoke and vaping appear to interfere with an infant's ability to regulate their breathing and make it harder for the baby to breathe properly. Smoking while pregnant and secondhand smoking can thus increase an infant's risk of SIDS.

Smoking also raises the risk of giving birth to a baby with birth defects. A massive study published in the journal *Human Reproduction Update* examined nearly fifty years of research on smoking and birth defects. The study examined about twelve million babies. Researchers looked closely at 172 scientific studies that have been published in the past few decades. Babies who were born to smokers were about a third more likely to have shortened or missing limbs. They were also about a third more likely to have a cleft lip or a cleft palate or have abnormally shaped heads or faces when compared to babies with mothers who did not smoke. Maternal smoking rates were also associated with about a 20 percent increased risk of conditions that can be dangerous and hard to fix such as gastrointestinal abnormalities that make it hard for babies to thrive and grow properly. Babies born to mothers who smoked were at also at vast risk of issues with the throat and the esophagus as well as the colon, intestine, the bile ducts, gallbladder, and the liver. Babies who were born to smokers also had a 50 percent greater chance of being born with their intestines hanging outside the body. Maternal smoking was also associated with a 20 percent increased risk of the baby being born with a blocked or a closed anus. Researchers examining the study also find a nearly 10 percent increased risk of heart defects. Boys were about 13 percent more likely to be born with undescended testes. Researchers aren't entirely sure of the mechanism that triggers these risks. They believe that as a mother smokes, she may be depriving her baby of oxygen as nicotine and carbon monoxide are both known to reduce the body's oxygen supply.

Some young women and teens may think that vaping is less harmful than smoking while pregnant. They may also be looking for ways to quit smoking and believe vaping will help them on this journey. E-cigs use an apparatus that turns chemicals found in cigarettes into a vapor that is inhaled rather than smoked. While this method means inhaling fewer chemicals into the body, e-cig users are still exposed to many known carcinogens and nicotine. Nicotine in any form is very dangerous to a developing fetus. Pregnant women who are thinking of quitting for the health of the baby should consult with a doctor. A doctor can suggest safe methods that can help stop smoking. Doing so can improve the odds of giving birth to a healthy baby and avoid exposing the newborn to the many risks of smoking when pregnant and secondhand smoke around the new baby.

22. Does smoking lead to the use of other drugs?

Habits tend to be formed early. A child may have a routine they follow after they get up each morning. As the child grows, they continue to follow the same pattern into adulthood. Habits take many forms. In many senses of the word, smoking is a habit. People have long wondered if smoking tobacco or marijuana can lead to the formation of other habits that can be equally, if not even more, detrimental. Gateway drugs are habit-forming drugs that may lead to the use of potentially more serious addictive narcotics. Over time, researchers believe that smokers may become more likely to use more serious drugs such as cocaine and heroin. While smoking is dangerous, it is still legal. Substances such as cocaine and heroin are not only extremely dangerous with many possible health complications. They're also illegal. Users or those who sell them can face long prison terms. Most smokers will not go on to use cocaine and heroin. Smoking does increase a smoker's chances of engaging in socially destructive behaviors. Nicotine can open the brain's doorway to addiction to other dangerous substances. Smoking can also make it harder for those searching for a way out of addiction to find a means to quit permanently.

Scientists have long known of the connection between smoking and the use other drugs. National surveys have indicated that nearly about nine in ten adult cocaine users have smoked cigarettes before they began to use cocaine. For researchers, the question was how and why nicotine exposure might make people potentially more vulnerable to cocaine addiction. A team from Columbia University with the help of the National Institute on Drug Abuse (NIDA) reported their results in *Science Translational Medicine*. They gave mice drinking water laced with nicotine for seven days. Scientists had previously found that a gene called *FosB* can initiate brain changes that make it more vulnerable to addiction and more likely that people will continue using cocaine over time. When mice were given water with nicotine, scientists found a 61 percent increase in the brain's expression or turning on of the *FosB* gene. After mice were given cocaine in addition to the nicotine, there was a 74 percent increase in *FosB* expression when compared to mice that were given cocaine alone. The mice model illustrates how it is possible that nicotine can increase a person's likelihood of becoming addicted to other drugs. Researchers believe it demonstrates how nicotine can shove aside some of the body's normal defenses and prime it to embrace potential addiction to cocaine.

Using nicotine can also make it harder for people to quit other addictions. A study in the *Journal of Clinical Psychiatry* looked at the connection between smoking and people who are attempting to rid themselves of addictions to cocaine and heroin. Over a three-year period, they examined data from about thirty-five thousand adults. Researchers found that both daily smokers and those who smoked less often were both at doubled risk of a drug relapse. Such odds continued to hold true even when researchers looked at other factors such as demographics and age and educational backgrounds. Those who began smoking during this time were also significantly more likely to relapse and begin using illicit substances again. Researchers believe that tobacco may become what scientists call a "cue" for the further use of such substances in that it reminds people how much they want to use the drugs. They also believe it indicates that the use of nicotine can increase the desire for opiates and make it more likely that users will return to them again even after they quit. Nonsmokers who began to smoke while part of the study were about five times as likely to indicate they were engaging in some form of illicit drug use compared with those who did not take up smoking at this time. Researchers also found that those who were able to quit smoking were also able to control their desire for illicit drugs during the study and that doing so "may even improve drug abstinence" and help them continue to avoid relapses over time.

Some teens today have begun to use e-cigs rather than traditional cigarettes or use them occasionally instead of using standard cigarettes. Teens and their parents may wonder if doing so makes it more likely that they'll use other kinds of drugs because they are using e-cigs. Findings published in the *New England Journal of Medicine* by Columbia professor of sociomedical sciences Denise Kandel and Nobel laureate Dr. Eric Kandel sought to examine the effects of e-cigs and find out if using e-cigs led users to smoke tobacco and use other drugs. Their study combines several disciplines such as epidemiology and molecular biology. Using mice models, they found that "e-cigarettes have the same physiological effects on the brain and may pose the same risk of addiction to other drugs as regular cigarettes." The authors further stated, "Nicotine clearly acts as a gateway drug on the brain, and this effect is likely to occur whether the exposure comes from smoking cigarettes, passive tobacco smoke, or e-cigarettes." They stated, "E-cigarettes may be a gateway to both combustible cigarettes and illicit drugs." Nicotine from e-cigs is still nicotine. It makes the brain more vulnerable to addiction to other substances. While not everyone will experience the same reaction, smoking tobacco or using e-cigs can lead to addiction and prevent people from shaking off long-term addiction problems.

23. Does chewing tobacco pose any special risks?

Tobacco has long been used in many varied ways across cultures and places. Some of the most popular today are smoking and chewing it. Chewing tobacco is quite common. It is sold in many parts of the United States. Many teens aren't sure if chewing tobacco poses the same health risks as smoking the substance. This form of tobacco use may seem less harmful than standard cigarettes and like chewing sugarless gum. Over the years, studies have found that chewing tobacco is not innocuous. Researchers have found many deleterious effects such as increasing the risk of many kinds of cancers. When left around the home, chewing tobacco can also create problems for younger household members.

There are lots of types of chewing tobacco on the market. Tobacco can be what is known as oral, chewing tobacco, or a form called spit tobacco. This kind of chewing tobacco is marketed in several forms. Chewing tobacco may be turned into plugs, bundles that are twisted, or just loose leaves that the chewer can chew in any amount. Dipping tobacco and snuff are another form of chewing tobacco that can be sold in dry or moist forms and with various added flavors. Moist snuff has been marketed as a less obvious way to use tobacco when with others. It typically comes in packages that look like tea bags. Dry snuff is on the market in powdered form intended to be used by sniffing it. In several Scandinavian countries, people commonly use snus. It usually has a flavored form that people hold in their mouths and then swallow the juice produced. Snus is similar to dissolvable tobacco. They take many forms including lozenges, pellets, strips, and other forms that can look a lot like candy and feel as appealing to small children. Dissolvable tobacco is also chewed or sucked as they slowly dissolve over time. Like snus, people swallow the resulting juice.

While burning tobacco in the form of smoke is the most dangerous form of tobacco use, chewing tobacco also poses specific risks that should not be underestimated. Like cigarette smoking, chewing tobacco also causes cancer. Chewing tobacco has over thirty chemicals that have been directly linked to cancer. When people chew tobacco, they get nicotine just like those who smoke it. Multiple types of cancer have been directly linked to chewing tobacco. Of particular note are cancers of the cheek, gum, mouth, pancreas, and tongue. It has also been linked to an increased risk of cancer of the esophagus. The more chewing tobacco you use, the greater risk of cancer.

Using chewing tobacco can also cause other health issues. Leukoplakias, also known as smoker's keratosis, are grayish-white patches that can form when people chew tobacco. They can be seen in the floor of the mouth, on the cheeks, or on the tongue. This is the body's reaction to chewing tobacco over a long period of time. Nicotine gets into the mucous membranes and causes irritation. While users will typically not feel any pain, it can be quite sensitive. The patches can lead to cancer. Those who stop using these forms of tobacco may find the patches will clear up on their own after they stop. However, a doctor may find early evidence of cancer in which case further treatment will be necessary. Smokeless tobacco can also stain the teeth and make them yellow. Users may also find that snuff and other smokeless tobacco products can harm their gums. Smokeless tobacco also has a relatively high sugar content. This can trigger cavities and ultimately cause lost teeth and bone.

Just as smoking tobacco has been linked to many kinds of other health problems, the same is true of smokeless tobacco. Like tobacco smoking, using chewing tobacco can also lead to high blood pressure and heart disease. Chewing tobacco also increases a user's risk of both heart attack and stroke as nicotine gets into their system and deprives cells of their ability to carry and use oxygen. Chewing tobacco can also affect the baby if pregnant. Moms who use smokeless tobacco are at risk of premature labor and stillbirth. Keeping smokeless tobacco in the home is also highly dangerous for young children. Packing methods can make it look very much like candy. Each year, many young children reach for chewing tobacco and get nicotine poisoning. Small doses of nicotine can cause poisoning and even kill young children. Pets can also get hold of chewing tobacco. Tobacco can harm your favorite kitten or beloved dog. Like users of cigarettes, those who chew tobacco can also become addicted to nicotine.

Even after spitting snuff out, there's still residual tobacco in the mouth that goes to the rest of the body and stays there. In fact, according to the National Cancer Institute, chewing tobacco keeps nicotine in the blood longer than smoking it. Many teens use smokeless tobacco and smoke tobacco as well. Doing so is highly dangerous and can vastly increase health risks over time.

Teens may think they use chewing tobacco as a way to help them quit smoking. However, chewing tobacco is also not for quitting smoking. Studies repeatedly indicate that users of smokeless tobacco are no more likely to quit smoking than those who do not. Using chewing tobacco alone may not satisfy the user's desire for nicotine and may even possibly increase it, leading to people smoking even more. Scientists and health officials know there is no form of safe tobacco use. Using snuff carries many of the same risks of smoking and may be equally hard to quit.

24. Can secondhand and thirdhand smoke pose health risks?

Secondhand smoking is smoke that gets in the body in one of two ways. People can be around someone as they exhale smoke. This is called mainstream smoke. People can also get exposed to secondhand smoke when there's a lit cigarette, e-cig, pipe, or other smoking delivery method near them. This is called sidestream smoking. Scientists call this form of smoke environmental tobacco smoke or ETS. It's also called passive smoking or involuntary smoking. While such actions would seem relatively harmless, over time health officials have in fact shown that secondhand smoking can pose serious health risks. When people are around tobacco smoke, they are inhaling it. Over time, it can damage the body in many of the same ways that tobacco does for someone who actively smokes.

Officials estimate that secondhand smoke has caused over two million deaths since the 1960s. Just like smokers, those exposed to secondhand smoke are at increased risk of many types of cancer. Secondhand smoke brings more than 7,000 chemicals into your lungs. Of these, about 70 are directly known to cause cancer. More than 250 are considered to be harmful. Every year, more than seven thousand people lose their lives to lung cancer because they have been exposed to secondhand smoke. If a husband or best friend smokes nearby, people are more likely to get diseases including brain cancer, bladder cancer, breast cancer, and stomach cancer. Secondhand smoking also causes heart disease. About thirty-five thousand people die prematurely each year from heart disease caused by smoking even if they never smoke a single cigarette. If exposed to second-hand smoke in the house or at the workplace, expect to increase that risk of heart disease by about a fourth compared to those who were not around sources of secondhand smoke. The same is true of the risk of a stroke. In any given year, more than eight thousand people will die from strokes just because they were around tobacco smoke. For those with a preexisting heart condition, it's especially important to stay away from secondhand smoke. According to the CDC, even "brief exposure" can interfere with the blood flow to the heart and cause a heart attack. Secondhand smoke may also have mental effects. Scientists believe it can increase rates of depression in nonsmokers.

Secondhand smoke harms babies and fetuses. Women exposed to secondhand smoke tend to go into labor earlier and have smaller babies as well as higher rates of stillbirths. After the baby is born, continuing to smoke puts the baby at risk from a condition called SIDS. This form of smoking is also highly dangerous for children. A child with a parent who smokes is more likely to get sick and get sick more often. They also have smaller lungs and are more vulnerable to conditions such as bronchitis and pneumonia that can scar their lungs as they grow up and make them likely to get such infections as adults. Children with asthma are particularly vulnerable if a parent smokes around them. Parental smoking can cause asthma attacks and make them both more severe and more frequent. Severe asthma attacks can kill. Children who have parents who smoke are also more in danger from ear infections. Chronic ear infections can damage the child's hearing permanently and cause speech delays that can interfere with their ability to learn. Health officials and scientists around the world believe that no amount of secondhand smoke is safe. Even a relatively short exposure time can result in dangerous and deadly effects such as triggering heart attacks and potentially deadly asthma attacks.

Dangers from smoking don't end when the smoking stops and the cigarette has been put out. The toxic chemicals found in tobacco smoke and vaping can linger on varied kinds of surfaces for months and even years. This is thirdhand smoking. Particles of nicotine and other dangerous chemicals from smoking in any form can settle on surfaces such as on tables and chairs and in the room's curtains. Chemicals can also linger on outdoor surfaces such as a building's windows and doors where smokers congregate. This kind of thirdhand smoke can also be found on shoes, gloves, scarves, and a bedspread. It may be in your favorite pair of jeans and the rug. It can also be found in the car and the patio where a friend comes over and starts to smoke. Over time, as the smoker smokes, more and more nicotine and other highly dangerous chemicals can accumulate where they've been smoking. It can even waft into your bedroom from a neighbor downstairs who opens a window and lets the smoke drift inside your bedroom. The stuff may smell badly and can turn whites dull.

Thirdhand smoking, like secondhand smoking, is also linked to a wide variety of health consequences. Even if you clean all areas where there was smoke present, the residue may still remain. It may create a cloud of toxic gas that is filled with substances that are known to cause cancer. Residue can get on skin, in the lungs, and into the digestive tract. A study in the journal *Tobacco Control* found that even if a smoker moved out and their homes were cleaned, there was thirdhand smoke residue in the lingering dust and home's surfaces. Thirdhand smoke has been shown to damage human DNA and impact the blood's ability to clot. Babies are especially at risk as they may put things covered in this residue in their mouths. This can increase a baby's lifetime exposure to the dangerous chemicals found in smoking and may increase their risks of the diseases that come with it.

25. Are certain forms of smoking, such as vaping and low-tar cigarettes, less dangerous?

Teens know smoking can have very negative effects on their health. A friend coughs a lot after a single cigarette. Another friend seems winded after a few hours at a party where there was a lot of smoking. Public health officials have been involved in governmental and global efforts to help make it easier to quit smoking and avoid smoking in the first place. While many teens are aware of these efforts, they may reason that certain forms of smoking such as vaping and low-tar cigarettes are not only less dangerous but may also pose few, if any, health risks at all. Over time, many such myths have developed around cigarettes and the kind of statements used on packaging as well as in marketing campaigns. One of the most common was the belief that certain types of cigarettes were less dangerous than other types of cigarettes. Cigarettes once had labels on them such as "low tar" or "light." This form of tobacco marketing developed in the 1960s and 1970s. The goal was an attempt to persuade smokers that some form of cigarette smoking was less dangerous than other kinds of cigarettes. In recent years, tobacco companies have gone even further. They brought out lines they called "ultra light" cigarettes or cigarettes that were supposed to be even less dangerous than the low tar and simply light versions. Tobacco companies argued that when they reduced the amount of tar in the cigarette, they were making it safer. Their cigarettes had holes in the filters that were thought to help trap tar, bring in more air to the smoker, and thus get rid of at least some of the dangerous chemicals found in cigarettes. In response, many smokers switched to these forms of cigarettes rather than deciding to quit smoking. In 2009, the Obama administration created the Family Smoking Prevention and Tobacco Control Act. This act empowers the Food and Drug Administration (FDA) to regulate many aspects of the tobacco industry both at home and abroad. One of the terms of the act was to give the administration the power to ban terms such as "light and low tar" when describing cigarettes unless FDA officials specifically decided otherwise. Officials have done so after numerous studies have indicated that even low-tar and light cigarettes can carry enormous health risks.

A research paper funded by the National Cancer Institute found that many tobacco companies have been able to get around this requirement. Instead of using terms such as "light and low tar," sub-brands are now referred to by colors such as blue, gold, and silver. Over nine out of ten smokers can still identify which sub-brands are intended to be low tar. Despite this relabeling, low-tar cigarettes and ultra lights are still just as dangerous as any other cigarettes. Studies have found that those who smoke such cigarettes are able to get around the lower tar feel by changing how they smoke. Smokers will typically take longer puffs on the cigarette. They'll also block the ventilation holes in the filter and often smoke more cigarettes. Such actions are designed to keep the body's level of nicotine use steady over time. One study of nearly a million Americans ultimately found that the level of tar made no difference in lung cancer deaths. Another study by the Ohio State University Comprehensive Cancer Center—Arthur G. James Cancer Hospital and Richard J. Solove Institute also looked at both cigarettes labeled light and ultra light. What they found was that smokers who smoked such cigarettes were at greater risk of another form of lung cancer called adenocarcinomas as they are taking deeper puffs and bringing more tobacco and other chemicals directly into their lungs. They are also equally likely to cause the same dangerous effects associated with standard cigarettes including an increased risk of heart attack and stroke as well as an increased risk of many types of cancers. As health officials have repeatedly stressed, there is no such thing as a safe cigarette.

Another form of smoking that has captured a great deal of attention in recent years is that of vaping and e-cigs. As stated in previous questions, these use a heater to heat fluid and turn them into a mist that people inhale. They may also take the form of a pod. Many teens tend to think this form of nicotine use is also harmless or at the very least does not carry significant health dangers. They may also think that using e-cigs can help them avoid addiction to standard cigarettes or help them quit. Such products have been marketed in this way in the past and continue to be marketed that way today. While e-cigs are a relatively recent development and an evolving form of nicotine use, data already in indicate that vaping also has some serious health risks just as smoking does. E-cigs still contain many of the same dangerous chemicals found in cigarettes. The nicotine found in e-cigs, just like the nicotine found in cigarettes, has been linked to many health issues. Even if it's not smoked, nicotine is still a dangerous substance. Users are more at risk from type II diabetes. Nicotine increases the heart rate and blood pressure, increasing chances of a heart attack and stroke. Nicotine also hurts brain development. When it does, the vaper may be left with decreased impulse control and attention deficit disorder and an impaired ability to respond to crucial life decisions needed as they grow up. Vaporizers also create problems by generating many of the same kinds of chemicals found in cigarettes such as formaldehyde that have detrimental effects even if you don't smoke. E-cigs are marketed in flavors that children find attractive. A small child may accidentally ingest the e-cig liquid from the pod and become dangerously ill. Older children may be tempted to try them because of such flavorings and ultimately wind up addicted to nicotine from a very early age. In addition, using e-cigs and vaping is not even associated with an increased ability to quit smoking. An article in the medical journal the *Lancet* examined multiple studies in attempting to find out if use of e-cigs had such a correlation. Researchers actually found that smokers who used e-cig users were actually less likely to quit smoking that those who did not use engage in vaping.

26. Can smoking kill me?

Smoking is the single biggest preventable cause of deaths worldwide. Six million people die each year because they smoke. They die from lung disease, heart disease, and other conditions, but they die because those conditions were directly triggered initially or made worse as a result of smoking. In the United States, about half a million people die each year because they smoke. The question is not if smoking can kill you. The question for the vast majority of smokers is how and why smoking will kill them. The process of smoking killing people begins early on from that very first intake of cigarette smoke. As the person smokes and continues to smoke, smoking can and does continue to impact their health. In teens, it kills the development of the lungs. Teens who begin smoking start before their lungs are fully developed and capable of full growth. A teen who begins smoking may never develop the same lung capacity as peers who did not smoke.

Smoking destroys the ability to taste, smell, see, hear, and touch. Smoking kills taste buds, making everything lack flavor. It also kills the cells of the nose, making it harder for smokers to smell properly. Smokers will find it harder to enjoy the delicate scent of a rose, appreciate the flavor of your grandmother's homemade tomato sauce, or grab a cup of coffee and the aromas it brings into the air. Smoking also kills eyesight. Studies have shown that smokers are three to four times as likely to develop AMD. Smokers are also more likely to develop other diseases of the eyes, including cataracts, glaucoma, and dry eye syndrome. Smokers are also in danger of killing parts of the body that bring sound to the brain. When people start smoking, chemical compounds in smoke interfere with the transmitters in the auditory nerves and make it less likely people can hear a full range of sounds. These chemicals can also irritate the lining of the middle ear, reducing the ability of that part of the ear to convey sound to the brain. Smokers may be prone to other conditions related to the degeneration of the ear such as painful ringing in the ear known as tinnitus. Smokers are also prone to repeated ear infections that can take a lot longer to heal. Over time, multiple ear infections can lead to gradual hearing loss. Teens who smoke also reduce their skin's ability to heal, leading to increased wrinkles and decreased skin sensitivity. Teens who smoke are more prone to get acne and more prone to get worse acne outbreaks, leading to scarring. Those who smoke will find they are at greater risk of a condition called Buerger's disease. This disease reduces the flow of blood to the arms and legs. Reach out for a comforting touch only to find there are areas of your skin that are not only numb but also aching and full of pain. Many of the same risks are true for those who vape and bring nicotine into their system each week.

While teens think smoking will not harm them if they are light or social smokers, studies show this to be false. Even a single cigarette in a day drastically increases the chances of dying much earlier. A study led by the National Cancer Institute in 2016 had a close look at people's smoking habits. About three hundred thousand people were asked to write about how often they smoked and how much. Part of the goal of the study was to help determine if light or social smoking can contribute to a person's overall risk of dying young. In the words of the team,

"Low-intensity smoking over the lifetime was associated with a significantly higher risk of all-cause mortality, including deaths from lung cancer and cardiovascular disease." Smoking what amounts to less than a single cigarette a day increased the risk of dying early by 64 percent. Those who smoked up to half a pack a day increased their chances of dying early by a whopping 87 percent compared to those who did not. Men who smoked just one cigarette in a day faced roughly half the risk of dying from stroke or heart attack that heavy smokers did. Women had about a third of the risk of heart attack and stroke as the heavy smokers. To put these numbers in perspective, just one cigarette a day can cut as much as ten to fifteen years off the smoker's life. Worse, it can compromise the quality of life years before you die. Even now, a cigarette a day can leave the smoker breathless, winded, and susceptible to all sorts of problems from colds to bronchitis and pneumonia. Just a few cigarettes now and then can also increase the risk of diabetes, just about every single kind of cancer, and diseases like lung cancer and arthritis. If the same number of teens continue to smoke, this means that over five million kids will die prematurely just because they smoked. That's about one in every thirteen of your peers.

There is hope. The same studies have also shown that smokers can reduce these risks drastically. Stop smoking before you're forty, and reduce that risk of dying by roughly 90 percent. Smoking is a greater cause of death than HIV, drug use, alcohol abuse, motor vehicle injuries, and death by firearms. You'll also reduce your risk of causing a fire in your home and destroying your senses. Smoking poses a greater risk to a girl's health than breast cancer. Smoke at an early age, and you're also more likely to abuse alcohol and engage in illicit drug taking. You're also sending a message to your peer group and your siblings. That message is that smoking is okay and will not harm them. This is why it's best to seek help with quitting as soon as you can. Your choice to walk away for good is one that can help your best friends, close relatives, and siblings follow the same path you do; avoid smoking forever, and add years to their life.

Tobacco Industry and Regulation

27. When did we discover the negative effects of smoking?

Teens today are aware that smoking is harmful. While it was obvious that smoking could have negative side effects, connections between smoking and ill health were not always easy to draw. It would take years of data and a great deal of medical investigation before doctors were able to firmly create a detailed picture of the negative effects of smoking. Much is known about how smoking can harm us today. Even more negative effects are still being discovered as doctors, scientists, and researchers continue to explore the tobacco plant. Using tobacco in some form was deeply popular in pre-Columbian America. Experts estimate that tobacco was first cultivated in the Peruvian highlands thousands of years ago. It rapidly spread across the entire Western Hemisphere and became part of many rituals. Tobacco was not perceived as harmful. Instead, it was an integral part of many ceremonial occasions. When Europeans encountered the Americas, they became aware of tobacco and nicotine use. By the middle of the sixteenth century, the Spanish, English, and French brought it back to Europe, where smoking and tobacco use quickly became embraced by many European rulers and large segments of the population. In the United States, tobacco was one of the largest cash crops grown for local use and exported to the Old World. For many years thereafter, a significant percentage of the population in the United States and many European nations used at least some form of tobacco each week. Men used it more often than women. The negative effects of tobacco on health began to be established early on. In the United States, esteemed physician Benjamin Rush argued that tobacco could be harmful and warned residents to avoid using it. Outdoor smoking was banned in Massachusetts in 1632 and on the streets of Philadelphia by the 1680s.

While only some people used tobacco, further developments began to make it more accessible to greater numbers. Technological developments during the Industrial Revolution created the means for tobacco makers to make larger quantities of ready-made cigarettes. Machines let tobacco companies go from a handful of rolled cigarettes each minute to over two hundred in the same time. Manufacturers realized they could gain even more customers with the use of advertising. In the United States alone, cigarette use climbed from forty-two million in 1875 to five hundred million just five short years later. Once cigarette smoking became so widespread, it was only a matter of time before the ill effects of smoking started to become ever obvious in the population at large. People began to notice that more people were dying earlier, and a significant percentage of them were heavy smokers. In response to the increasing availability of tobacco, state government officials began to restrict tobacco use. They focused largely on the age of the consumer. While smoking was becoming more common, it started to really take off during World War II. As part of their promotional efforts, tobacco companies were allowed to provide soldiers with cigarettes, making them a popular item soldiers could use on their own or trade for other items. This was also part of a tobacco industry effort to fight against regulations that governed tobacco sales. In fact, tobacco marketing was so successful that cigarette manufacturers were able to convince many companies to drop any age-related restrictions on tobacco sales. The following decade saw increased marketing not only to men but to women as well. Both sexes were encouraged to see smoking as a form of liberation against social norms and a modern form of recreation. Women were especially encouraged to see tobacco as a means of keeping their appetite suppressed in order to adhere to the lean and boyish silhouettes of the day. Such efforts worked for the companies as the numbers of female smokers rose by one-third in a single decade. Smoking continued to gain popularity both in the United States and Europe as tobacco companies kept the same strategy of providing soldiers with tobacco during World War II.

The Surgeon General's Report

Once smoking became a part of life for many people, doctors started to notice side effects from tobacco use. British doctors linked snuff to nose cancer in 1791. By 1912, a tenuous connection between lung cancer and smoking began to be established. In the coming decades, doctors, public health officials, and specialists in epidemiology made connections between smoking and diseases such as lung cancer. Once a rarity, by 1950, lung cancer overtook all other cancers and became the most commonly diagnosed cancer in American men. It was during this decade that five large studies were published. Each one linked the explosion in lung cancer cases with the rise in the number of smokers. The definitive study looked at over a hundred and fifty thousand American men between the ages of fifty and sixty-nine. The authors published a historic study in the *Journal of the American Medical Association* in 1954. The study made the definitive assertion that men who smoked had a far higher death rate than men who did not. By 1957, the American surgeon general told the American public it was the official position of the U.S. Public Health Service that there was enough evidence to indicate a positive relationship between smoking and lung cancer. The original study was followed up by an even larger study of over a million Americans in 1959. It was called Cancer Prevention Study I, and it further established the ill effects of smoking on health. In 1961, multiple major American public health groups including the American Cancer Society and the National Tuberculosis Association sent a letter to President Kennedy. They urged him to have a greater look at the dangers of smoking. Kennedy responded by forming a national advisory committee headed by his surgeon general to look at the issue of smoking dangers in greater detail. For more than a year, the members of the board examined many studies, spoke to health experts, and looked at data collected in five separate nations over the course of nearly twenty years. One hundred and fifty experts had a close look at over seven thousand articles. Their careful examination led to a seminal moment in the history of American medicine, the history of tobacco use, and one of the most important conclusions ever produced and confirmed.

Published on January 11, 1964, the study immediately made instant front-page news in the United States and the rest of the globe. Called *Smoking and Health: Report of the Advisory Committee to the Surgeon General*, it made many huge important conclusions about the effects of smoking on people's health and well-being. The surgeon general's report ultimately argued that smokers had a 70 percent higher risk of death when compared with nonsmokers. The report also asserted that smokers had a nine- to tenfold risk of lung cancer when compared to those who did not smoke. The surgeon general also linked smoking to conditions such as chronic bronchitis, emphysema, and coronary heart disease. The writers also linked smoking to lower birth weights in newborns. The aftermath of the report had a major effect on public attitudes toward cigarette use. The following year, Congress required all packs of cigarettes to carry a warning indicating the findings of the report. By 1970, cigarette television and radio advertising had been banned in the United States. The report also sparked additional public and private sector efforts to continue to investigate the possible negative effects of smoking. These efforts continue to this day.

28. Why is smoking legal?

Smoking has almost no health benefits. As soon as you inhale, you start to make it harder to breathe. You make it harder to run, you fill your clothing with layers of toxic chemicals, and you increase your chances of bronchitis. Continue to smoke, and you'll rapidly up your risks of everything from cancers to hearing loss, heart attack, and stroke. Smoke, and you will increase your chances of an early death and your risks of serious, chronic medical conditions. Continue smoking over time, and you'll lose thousands of dollars and expose everyone around you to the dangers of secondhand and thirdhand smoke. Given such known health problems, you might be wondering why smoking is still legal. From hard drugs to driving without a seat belt, many other comparable behaviors are illegal in the United States. So why is something with as many known risks and absolutely no real benefit still allowed in this country? Many factors go into keeping smoking legal. This includes the fact that smoking has deep roots in the United States as well as the popularity of this substance and the history of movements such as Prohibition that made alcohol consumption illegal in the United States in the 1920s. Rather than an outright ban, government officials have chosen to work to reduce overall smoking rates over time. This policy has been yielding results as the number of teen smokers has dropped and continues to drop in this country. Unfortunately, companies have been fighting back by finding ways to hook new smokers. New developments like e-cigs threaten to undo decades of anti-smoking and antinicotine and tobacco use efforts.

Smoking bans have been in place in many places as early as the sixteenth century. Mexican Catholics were banned from smoking. Other laws and efforts followed suit as smoking spread to Europe. Smoking was banned in the Ottoman Empire and parts of Austria as well as New Zealand and certain Canadian provinces. In the United States, roughly half of all American states had banned tobacco sales to minors by 1890.

As early as 1880, several states, including New Jersey, New York, Michigan, and Oregon, banned tobacco sales to anyone under sixteen. By the turn of the century, several states, including North Dakota, Iowa, and Washington, banned the sale of cigarettes altogether. During the 1920s, all states but two had regulations restricting cigarette sales to minors. Yet this did not stop people from using tobacco in other forms. About 80 percent of all American men had at least a cigar a day. Sales of cigars had reached six billion by the turn of the last century. Multiple other bans began to evolve as well. These bans were fought by the tobacco industry. Since that time, other kinds of smoking restrictions have been in place. Restaurants and other private spaces have been required to create both smoking and nonsmoking areas in many states. Smoking has also been banned outright by many legislators in places ranging from public parks to schools. Certain colleges, such as Indiana University, ban all smoking on campus. Others, such as Perdue University and Rutgers, allow smoking only in certain parts of the campus. State governments, including Colorado and Michigan, have enacted a statewide smoking ban. This ban means that smoking is banned in all indoor spaces including workplaces. In some of our largest cities such as New York, smoking is not allowed in nearly all outdoor spaces such as parks, public beaches, and pedestrian plazas. Many more states and local municipalities are expected to follow the same path and enact restrictions on smoking in places such as public transportation, hospitals, and other areas where people live and work. E-cigs as well as vaping are also being banned in many places right now.

While laws have been set in motion gradually, some may wonder why Congress has not enacted a national statewide smoking ban. Historically, Americans have resisted pressure from Congress and the White House. The national government sets policy in many areas ranging from foreign policy to domestic affairs. Under the Obama administration, further laws governing the use of tobacco were set in place in 2009. The administration gave the U.S. Food and Drug Administration (FDA) the right to regulate how tobacco products are manufactured, marketed, and distributed. The Tobacco Control Act has many provisions, including regulations that require tobacco companies to list all the ingredients in cigarettes. Companies are also not allowed to advertise to teens. The act ultimately establishes what it calls appropriate protection of public health. These regulations represent some of the many restrictions that are likely to continue on the sale, advertising, and distribution of all tobacco products. Efforts at regulation of e-cigs and vaping also continue. FDA officials have begun attempts to investigate issues related to e-cigs and vaping in more detail. New laws are expected to come down the pipeline that should ideally help reduce the number of teens who are using such products and help them quit for good. As history shows, it can take time for health officials to act in response to new products on the market even when such products are obviously dangerous.

29. How is tobacco regulated around the world?

Tobacco use is a concern not only in the United States. Officials estimate that smoking is directly responsible for 10 percent of all deaths globally. Given that these deaths are totally preventable, this makes smoking an issue of concern for global health experts in every country. Some countries regulate smoking heavily. Others regulate smoking lightly, if at all. Just as some states ban smoking in some areas, the same is true with a varied patchwork of regulations across the globe. One nation, Bhutan, completely bans the sale and production of all tobacco-related products. This is rare. In many nations, especially many poor nations, smoking remains part of the local culture. It is essentially sanctioned socially as well as by government officials who loathe to confront ingrained customs even in the name of protecting public health. Bhutan was the first country in the entire world to go totally smoke free. Information on cigarette use across the world can be hard to find as it may not be considered a problem. The World Health Organization (WHO) has taken a leading role in efforts to reduce tobacco use and consumption. Under the details of the WHO Framework Convention on Tobacco Control in 2003, the WHO implemented the world's first public health treaty. This treaty, signed by more than 180 countries, has multiple provisions. Signees agree to engage in multiple regulatory efforts against tobacco use. These include tobacco taxes, bans on tobacco advertising, efforts to ban smoking from the workplace, the creation of spaces free from tobacco smoke, and warnings on tobacco industry products. Still, the WHO reports that such regulations are not always honored. In fact, according to WHO reports, "more than half of the world's population lives in areas that lack even minimally adequately recent information on tobacco use." People in many nations across the globe are forced to endure tobacco use in many places such as hospitals and parks. Kids even need to put with smoking at school in many places even if they have allergies or other medical conditions that might be made worse by smoking. Of the world's population, only about one in twenty people live in an area where they have any basic right of access to smoke-free spaces at all. Many countries barely regulate tobacco use. Seventy-four percent of the world's population live in a nation where it is legal to smoke in a healthcare facility even around pregnant women and babies. Roughly eight in ten children and teens live in nations that still allow smoking in educational institutions, including kindergartens, grade schools, high schools, and universities, both public and private. Two-thirds of the world's population live in countries that allow smoking in all indoor spaces, including government offices, bars, restaurants, and private companies in all industries. This means that workers have no protection against others who choose to smoke. Like teens, they must work in conditions that expose them to the effects of smoking by other people.

In countries where tobacco use is regulated, such regulations may not be enforced. A mere sixteen countries have laws that cover the right to totally smoke-free workplaces, schools, parks, and other public and private spaces. The WHO states that only a third of these nations enforce existing laws with any frequency. Countries like Uganda and Niger have laws on the books, but few law enforcement officials are willing to empower people with their right to a smoke-free environment. Other countries have such laws and do their best to enforce them. As of 2004, Ireland does not allow smoking in spaces ranging from bars to parks. Nations as diverse as Italy, Norway, Canada, Italy, and Uruguay all crack down on smoking. Access to efforts to help people quit is often equally restricted. Only forty-four nations offer resources that smokers need to permanently quit. Some nations have been providing subsidies. Brazilian officials have implemented many different forms of help including subsidized nicotine patches and a quit line staffed by experts. Similar efforts have been made by officials in the United Kingdom.

Another area that is often skirted by country officials is that of advertising. Advertising is a particularly crucial outlet for tobacco companies. Tobacco ads accomplish goals such as establishing a brand image and bringing in new clients. Banning advertising has been shown to reduce the ability of companies to expand into new markets and create a favorable image of smoking in the public mind. While bans against advertising are on the books in over a hundred countries, they are rarely enforced. In many nations, tobacco companies are freely allowed to advertise on the internet as well as in print media and on television. Tobacco companies are also allowed to sponsor sports teams and place logos on clothing. Tobacco taxes are another area where government officials could choose to discourage tobacco use. Placing taxes on tobacco use, according to the *Tobacco Atlas*, is a very efficient method of reducing consumption of tobacco products. Unfortunately, they are rarely used. Some nations, such as the United States and New Zealand, impose relatively heavy tobacco taxes. Four in ten people live in countries where tobacco taxes are minimal at best. In countries like China and Indonesia, this means that the price of a pack of cigarette can be less than two dollars. That's expensive compared to local incomes but still within fiscal reach of much of the population. This is well below the cost that tobacco consumption places on society. Cheaper tobacco prices are one way that tobacco companies hook people on smoking and keep them smoking for life. Even these small sums can be hard on poor people in developing countries where yearly consumption of tobacco products can consume as much as 10 percent of a household's income. Only a small fraction of the world lives in a society that taxes tobacco products to make up for the real cost of the product. This small fraction is unfortunately among the few groups of people that have schools, parks, workplaces, and other gathering places where they are not exposed to secondhand or thirdhand smoke.

Laws about vaping follow similar patterns worldwide. Some nations have banned the practice, while many others have not. A number of countries ban the sales of e-cigs and vaping equipment but do not ban people from possessing e-cigs and vaping items. Some country officials not only ban e-cigs but also imprison travelers for importing them. Bring an e-cig to Thailand, and you might face imprisonment and fines. The same is true in Taiwan. Government officials in nations from Mexico to the Philippines have also imposed similar restrictions. Other nations have a varied mix of differing regulations. Canada has banned vaping for those under nineteen. In India, some states allow vaping and e-cigs, while others ban them completely. Given the increasing evidence that vaping and the use of e-cigs are just as dangerous as the use of other smoking-related products, it is likely that more restrictions and total bans on the use of these forms of nicotine use will continue. It is also likely that officials in other parts of the world will respond to efforts by companies that promote vaping and the use of e-cigs by not necessarily enforcing such regulations.

30. How big is the tobacco industry?

The marketing and selling of tobacco products began several hundred years ago. Since tobacco was brought from the New World to the Old, it has caught on and become part of the culture of commerce. Planters took advantage of this growing market to create a cash crop they grew in America and shipped to the American public and an awaiting European audience. The process of growing, creating, and selling tobacco products still continues today. Tobacco use and consumption are now spread across the world. Of all the world's crops, tobacco is one of the globe's most profitable ones. Revenues from tobacco and sales of e-cigs are about $700 billion annually. This makes it one of the biggest industry sectors worldwide and an incredibly lucrative one. While cigarette use is gradually declining in high-income nations, it is increasing even more in middle- and low-income parts of the world. Tobacco companies are increasingly shifting their marketing efforts from countries where restrictions are in place to countries that lack them. Cigarette companies are chasing after new markets in Asia and Africa. Growing populations combined with almost nonexistent restrictions on smoking have made such areas a prime target for market penetration and expansion. Sales in Asia, the Middle East, and Africa have grown in the past two decades, while sales in every other region on the globe have started to decline and are likely to continue to do so in the coming years. The same is true for the use of e-cigs.

Another trend in tobacco sales that is also likely to continue is the creation of huge, transnational cigarette companies with global reach and even more clout. At the turn of this century, about 40 percent of all global tobacco sales were controlled by only five companies. Fifteen years later, those same companies now control about 80 percent of the global tobacco markets. The five companies that have largely cornered the market for tobacco span several countries. Philip Morris is perhaps the best-known company, with headquarters in Switzerland. It only sells tobacco products outside of the United States. Philip Morris also holds about 35 percent of JUUL sales, thus making it arguably the largest marketing of e-cigs in the United States. The company has about 14 percent of the world cigarette market and a greater percentage of the e-cig market. China National Tobacco Corporation is owned by the Chinese government. The company has the lion's share of the growing Chinese market and illustrates part of the reason why the Chinese government refuses to engage in concerted efforts to reduce smoking. It controls about 37 percent of the world tobacco market and brings in about $90 billion annually. British American Tobacco is a London-based company and the world's third-largest tobacco marketer. It is the world's largest publicly traded tobacco company and has profits of about $4 billion yearly. This situation has not gone unnoticed by governments where it does business. Several seek to hold it responsible for the damage done by the promotion of tobacco consumption. British American Tobacco has been sued by many governments, including those of Canada and Nigeria, for deliberately attempting to encourage smoking.

The company operates in over two hundred markets around the world, including Bangladesh and the Gulf states. Japanese Tobacco markets to smokers in Japan and the rest of the world. One-third of the company's shares are held by the Japanese government, creating a situation similar to that in China. It is probably part of the reason why smoking restrictions are not as strict in this part of the world compared to government antismoking campaigns in other highly developed nations. The Imperial Tobacco Group is a British company that operates in many global markets and produces many kinds of tobacco products such as cigars and rolling papers. Five nations compromise more than half of the global smoking marketplace. The top five nations for profits are China, Indonesia, Russia, the United States, and Japan. Other important nations for tobacco profits are Turkey, Egypt, Bangladesh, India, and Germany. Cigarette sales continue to grow in China even as they are decreasing in other parts of the world. This is an over $200 billion market. India is another country with a population comparable in size to China. Smokeless tobacco and hand-rolled products have helped make this a major target market for worldwide cigarette makers.

Even with restrictions and lawsuits, the tobacco industry continues to generate massive profits. The combined profits from the largest tobacco companies are about $35 billion. To put that in perspective, that's more than the profits earned by industry giants like McDonald's and Microsoft. If tobacco were a nation, it would have an income larger than many nations including Cameroon, Estonia, and Madagascar. These are profits that accrue solely to the manufacturers. Meanwhile, American taxpayers are on the hook for thirty-five dollars per pack. The costs of caring for smoking in Egypt consume over 10 percent of the nation's health-care budget. In China, smoking kills over a million people each year. Smokers spend nearly $200 billion in health-care costs in the United States annually. The costs of smoking reverberate all over the economy in the United States and other nations. American smokers can expect to earn only 80 percent as much as coworkers who don't smoke. Start smoking before twenty-four, and that wage penalty will start to hit you even before you hit the job market. You don't have to smoke all that much. The penalty is much the same whether you smoke a pack a day or just a single cigarette. You'll also suffer with increased costs in other ways. Many insurance companies, including health insurance and car insurance companies, charge smokers more than those who don't light up. Tobacco companies are essentially earning huge profits all over the world while passing the real costs of their products to the consumers. Much the same is true of e-cigs and vaping. JUUL Labs is valued in excess of

$30 billion, making it one of the world's most profitable companies. Experts estimate sales of several billion dollars yearly. Company officials anticipate expansion into other markets in other parts of the world, making it even more lucrative even in the face of crackdowns on the sale of vaping and e-cigs in other nations.

31. How is tobacco advertised?

Advertising is an ancient process that can be used to introduce consumers to new products, increase brand awareness, and create a favorable public image. People see products advertised and tend to remember them. They want you to see products and associate them with highly positive qualities such as youth, vigor, beauty, and wealth. The same is true of tobacco companies. Tobacco companies have been making use of advertising to introduce people to their products' allegedly superior qualities for many hundreds of years. Today, even as tobacco advertising is heavily restricted in the United States and many other countries, tobacco companies still find ways to reach out to the public and imply that smoking is a desirable activity. Smoking cigarettes really began to take off in the United States in the aftermath of the Civil War. It was at that point that mechanization began to make it far easier to take tobacco and turn it into cigarettes that more people could afford. It was also at this point that cigarette advertising really began in earnest. Prior efforts focused largely on the use of snuff and tobacco to put in a man's pipe. New forms of advertising used various media to connect with customers and aimed to let them distinguish one brand from another. With the rise of the department store in the 1850s, store owners sought to draw in customers. One of their favored methods was to give out colorful paper cards. These cards, known as trading cards, were also used by manufacturers of everything from chocolates to detergents. By the 1880s, tobacco companies decided it was time to join them. Cards were designed in vivid colors and meant to be collected. They were also there to prevent the cigarettes inside from being squashed. Popular card images included women in bathing costumes and sports heroes. Honus Wagner, a baseball player for the Pittsburgh Pirates and a non-smoker, objected to having his picture on the card. It was withdrawn and now commands lots of money when put up for auction. These cards also featured many other images, from Shakespearean quotes to chess problems. They proved so popular that children asked adults leaving tobacco shops for the cards in order to trade them with others. The cards continued to be a huge way to advertise tobacco products until World War II.

In the 1990s, health officials sought to revive the cards in order to warn teens and adults about the dangers of smoking while mocking smoking companies at the same time.

The 1920s and 1930s were the heyday of print cigarette advertising. These ads appear quite startling today. Full-page advertisements in vivid colors in some of America's most popular magazines were common. Even odder to the modern eye, ads often featured doctors extolling the virtues of smoking. While some doctors suspected smoking might be dangerous, the vast majority believed that no such connection existed. Many doctors were smokers. Tobacco company officials used all sorts of statements from doctors to imply that their products were safe. Philip Morris, a leading tobacco manufacturer then and one of the major investors in JUUL, used print media and doctors to repeatedly imply that its brand of cigarettes was safer than other brands. Companies also sought to link developments in science and medicine to smoking in their print advertising. One brand even advertised that more doctors smoked their brand than any other brand. Radio advertisements were also popular during this period as was advertising on television. Smoking was featured in many television shows and programs. These two outlets remained quite popular with cigarette makers until tobacco companies were banned from using them in 1970 by the Public Health Cigarette Smoking Act. Commercials exhorting people to smoke were replaced by public service ads that urged people never to start as well as providing publicly funded resources for those seeking to quit.

Despite the many contemporary limitations on smoking advertising, tobacco company executives find ways to reach customers with advertising. Health officials estimate tobacco companies spend billions of dollars to market cigarettes and smokeless tobacco products. Most of their marketing efforts in the United States have taken three forms. One of the biggest is giving stores rebates for the cost of the retail price of their products. The net effect is reducing the price per pack to consumers even in the face of often stiff state and local tobacco taxes. Lower prices are a form of advertising in that it makes it easier for consumers to purchase that initial pack. Once they buy that first pack, many will go on to become repeat customers. In essence, this is a form of discounting that is directly designed to mask the real costs that smoking imposes on the smoker and society at large. Such payments typically account for about $7 billion annually. Another form of financing and advertising that tobacco companies use to increase sales and increase different cigarette brands' visibility to customers are direct payments to retailers to stock and display specific brands in their stores. Costs for this program typically run over

$200 million annually. Tobacco companies also entice retailers to stock and display their products with the use of in-store promotions, rebates for selling a certain amount in a given quarter, and other forms of pricing discounts. According to the American Lung Association, a 10 percent increase in the cost of cigarettes leads to a 7 percent reduction in the number of teens who smoke. Tobacco companies also make specific efforts to attract certain minority communities and women. Companies have sponsored Chinese and Vietnamese festivals such as New Year's celebrations as well as supporting Asian American businesses. In the African American communities, cigarette companies have purchased many large billboards and other easily visible signage. A 2007 study found that such signs were about two and a half times more common in African American neighborhoods than in neighborhoods with comparable demographics. Tobacco companies are also using other forms of media such as popular teen internet websites. Many media platforms such as Snapchat have fought back with bans on tobacco company advertising. Such bans are only expected to continue even as tobacco companies look for ways to evade them.

The marketing and advertising of e-cigs have been just as bold. JUUL, in particular, has used mass media outlets to reach out to teens in ways that are not allowed by traditional cigarette and tobacco manufacturers. As a nicotine delivery method, officials face far fewer restrictions on advertising methods. Experts at Stanford University examined the methods used by JUUL to reach out to clients. The company ostensibly began as a method to help adult smokers quit. Researchers found that "in the summer of 2015, Juul's product launch coincided with sampling events in major US cities." According to Stanford University research, "Good-looking young people distributed free JUULs at movie and music events." Here, the "principle focus of these activities was to get a group of youthful influencers to accept gifts of Juul products" and then "to try out their various flavors, and then to popularize their products among their peers." Company officials made a deliberate effort to borrow from popular cigarette advertising methods. They used bright colors and images of young people enjoying the product. They also took to Instagram and worked with social influencers to help make the product known. Multiple hashtags such as "#juul, #juulvapor, #switchtojuul, #vaporized" were used as promotional tools. Katy Perry was even shown using JUUL at the Golden Globes. It was not until several years later in 2018, in part from pressure from the FDA, that company officials switched to the ostensible promotion of the product as a means of quitting smoking. Early market penetration efforts that were free of traditional restrictions on smoking-related products allowed the company to reach out to teens and establish a following.

---❖---

Quitting

32. How addictive is smoking?

Addiction is a highly complicated condition. Over time, addictions create emotional, mental, physical problems in sufferers. Yet people continue to use such substances. In general, an addiction is a craving for a substance that people find hard to overcome. A person can be addicted to many things including alcohol and illicit drugs. People become addicted for a great many reasons. Some people have an inborn tendency to become addicted that shows up even with limited exposure. A person's addiction can be triggered by many things. For many sufferers, it shows up once exposed to outside pressures and stressful situations such as a childhood spent in a dangerous neighborhood. Addiction can also develop when people are exposed to the availability of certain substances or when people are part of peer groups that engage in such behaviors. Many different types of chemical compounds can trigger addictive behavior in users.

As so many medical studies across varied global populations have demonstrated, smoking is extremely addictive. Smokers are exposed to addictive substances when they light up or chew tobacco. The active ingredient that is known to cause addiction is nicotine. Nicotine has literally been shown to alter the structure of the brain and make it hard to quit. Most smokers are well aware of the effects of smoking on their lives and would like to quit. Nicotine is so addictive that users find it nearly impossible without repeated tries. Two out of three smokers would like to quit. While half attempt to do so each year, most will not succeed without dedicated outside help. Many people require upwards of half a dozen efforts at quitting only to find they keep going back to smoking. The primary reason they find it so hard is because of an addiction to nicotine. Nicotine impacts how you feel, see the world, and think. It shapes your body's responses and leads to a daily routine that revolves around getting a nicotine fix. Changes that nicotine introduces can be permanent. Many people are surprised to learn that varied studies by the Centers for Disease Control and Prevention (CDC) have found nicotine to be just as addictive as alcohol and even cocaine. In the United States, it is the most common addiction. Using nicotine creates separate receptors in the brain just for nicotine. These receptors want to get that substance again and again as it release a chemical called dopamine that can lead to feelings of pleasure. When people light up, they get access to nicotine in short bursts. People feel temporarily happy. This sense fades quickly, leaving the body craving ever more nicotine just to feel that same feeling of pleasure. People find they need to smoke more just to feel the same way. When they try to quit, the craving for nicotine becomes incredibly hard to overcome as it has become hardwired in the structure of the brain. Worse still, quitting can lead to unpleasant emotional symptoms that can lead to changes in personality and ability to cope with daily life tasks. A smoker may feel depressed, anxious, and irritable as well as find it hard to concentrate. Smokers attempting to quit find they are prone to responding inappropriately at work, at school, and in social situations. A smoker may also experience other physical symptoms such as insomnia, headaches, abdominal cramps, and increased appetite. Such feelings can become serious for a few days and then gradually start to taper off. For some, these symptoms can linger for weeks and impact all areas of their life, tempting the smoker to go back to smoking.

Scientists used to think that it was necessary to smoke at least five cigarettes a day in order to become addicted to nicotine. However, a study in the *Archives of Pediatric and Adolescent Medicine* found that, for a significant percentage of the population, smoking even a single cigarette can saturate the brain's nicotine receptors and alter the function and structure of the brain. Over time, the smoker begins to crave more nicotine. Changes in the brain caused by smoking can also continue for years even if the smoker can quit. The same changes were seen in those who chewed tobacco rather than smoked it. In one in ten teens, a single cigarette led to addiction. It took only a few more to lead to addiction in a quarter of the teens studied. Many smokers take about ten puffs for every single cigarette they smoke. These puffs go directly into the brain. A pack of cigarettes typically contains twenty-five cigarettes. That means two hundred and fifty hits of nicotine that then release dopamine in the brain. A significant number of teens who vape find vaping isn't enough to deliver the amount of nicotine they crave. Many turn to regular cigarettes. The brain has been primed by the vaping to want more of the nicotine that the cigarette delivers. Even minor exposure to a short burst of nicotine from any source can ultimately lead people to become addicted to smoking. The vast amount of nicotine found in a single pod is equivalent to a pack of cigarettes. Users often smoke and vape in the course of a single smoking cession.

33. What is quitting cold turkey? Is it effective?

You may have heard of the term "quitting cold turkey." This phrase means someone has decided to completely and abruptly stop smoking and the use of all other nicotine-containing products. Smokers who quit cold turkey do not seek any outside help or support such as nicotine gum or help with a support group or counseling by medical experts. In theory, it sounds easy. In practice, however, many smokers find quitting cold turkey really hard. Experts estimate that less than 10 percent of all smokers are able to quit without some form of assistance. Thomas Glynn, director of cancer science and trends at the American Cancer Society, compares quitting cold turkey to attempting to walk across a tightrope without a net. It's understandable that people want to quit under their own terms. They want to be free to decide exactly when they're going to quit and how they're going to do it. At the same time, the pull that nicotine has on the human mind and body is intense. Most smokers underestimate the reality of nicotine addiction and how hard it is to move past it. When people stop smoking, they are likely to experience short-term effects that can be hard to manage. Someone choosing to quit cold turkey may find in the days following their decision they are irritable with friends, angry at school, and less able to cope with stress. Quitting smoking instantly leaves your body without a buffer to help reduce such feelings. This is why many smokers may attempt to quit cold turkey several times only to return to smoking again.

Choosing the cold turkey route can work for some people. It's important to keep in mind that every single smoker has a different set of circumstances that might make this choice work for them. Some smokers find that toughing it out during this period lets them focus on quitting smoking to the exclusion of all else. Setting aside a specific time frame to cope with this problem will get past it. Those who've been down this road before know what to expect and may have developed strategies that can help them maintain awareness and keep to their goal of quitting smoking. Some people have a wide social support network. Friends and family can help the smoker quit cold turkey. A friend can share their own experiences and cheer the smoker on as they attempt to become an ex-smoker. Close family members can also help by being patient and understanding that the smoker is facing a difficult challenge they hope to overcome permanently. Many people choose to let others know they are planning to quit smoking in advance in order to warn them about any sudden changes in their behavior. Picking the cold turkey route has a few advantages. Other quitting smoking methods require funds, time, and commitment. The smoker does not need to head to scheduled counseling appointments or spend money on quitting smoking methods. While this form of smoking cessation can be effective and inexpensive, it's important to begin the process carefully. Most people fail because they do not make a plan to see it through. Making a detailed plan before you begin will up your chances of shaking off an addiction to nicotine. It's a good idea to pick a specific day a few days in advance. A weekend day or when you're on school break lets you do other things during that time frame that can help you focus on other activities. Clear out all smoking-related items from your home and other places like your locker and a part-time job. If you have peers who smoke or vape, you might try to avoid meeting with them while you're in the process of quitting. Avoid places you know they hang out. It's also a good idea to lay in a supply of items that you can put in your mouth. Chewing gum, breath mints, and anything else that you like to eat slowly can help. Water is another good thing to keep on hand. Place a few bottles in the freezer, and bring them with you throughout the day. A water bottle can be stowed away in your backpack. Other ways to occupy your mouth and stay hydrated include hot soup in the winter and fruit drinks when it's hot outside. Staying active and getting lots of exercise can also be useful when you're trying to quit. Create a list of benefits that you'll get from not smoking, and keep it on hand to look at. If cold turkey doesn't work, bear in mind you can always get help from others to say goodbye to nicotine for good. These same strategies can be applied if you are attempting to quit using e-cigs.

34. If I'm smoking only one or two cigarettes a day, do I really need to quit?

Smoking is like many other human activities. Some people smoke a lot. They might have upwards of a pack a day. Others may grab only a single cigarette or two a day and then a few more on weekends. Smokers who smoke only a few cigarettes each week engage in what is known as light smoking. A light smoker, unlike a heavy smoker, is someone who tends to smoke less than many of their peers. About a quarter of smokers only have a handful of cigarettes or even avoid smoking completely most of the time unless under certain circumstances. This form of smoking is indeed better for you than smoking a pack or more each day. If you smoke only intermittently or smoke only e-cigs, you might be wondering if you need to stop altogether. Light smoking is better for your overall health than heavy smoking. But, like all forms of nicotine and tobacco use, the best thing to do is quit completely. Like other forms of smoking, even light smoking is dangerous. For a long time, those who studied smoking believed that this kind of smoking pattern could help people by letting them gradually taper down their use of cigarettes and eventually become nonsmokers. Instead, many people continue to be light smokers for many years. Rather than quit, they still have a smoking dependency. This form of smoking also tends to be underestimated by people who study smoking. When asked if they smoke, many people who actually are light smokers will tell researchers they don't smoke at all. They may not consider using e-cigs a form of smoking. The underlying presumption many make is they're not really smokers unless they're heavy smokers. As a result, they might not get the help they need to figure out how to drop the habit. Even if you smoke or use e-cigs only a little, you should quit as soon as you can.

Light smokers are still in danger. A study published in the *British Medical Journal* looked closely at studies examining the behavior of millions of smokers over time. The comprehensive study examined over 140 studies in great detail from 21 countries. These studies were conducted between 1946 and 2015, making it possible to follow five million smokers over time and see what happened. Their findings were startling. Light up once a day, and increase your chances of having a heart attack by 48 percent. You'll also up the risk of a stroke by 25 percent. That's just for men. Women face even greater risks from social smoking. A single smoke a day increases the risk of a heart attack by 51 percent and stroke by 37 percent. Researchers anticipated that smoking only one cigarette a day would have only 5 percent the risk of smoking an entire pack. Not so. Men were at risk from smoking by over 40 percent with a single daily cigarette. Women faced risks of over 30 percent. Researchers examined the data in even greater detail. They pulled out data that took out people with conditions that predisposed them to heart attack and stroke, such as high blood pressure, obesity, diabetes, and how much exercise people got. The results remained the same. Just one cigarette break a day was enough to continue to increase the smoker's risk of getting heart disease or suffering a stroke. That's clear data that indicate that it is best for even so-called light smokers to stop smoking as soon as they can. One of the issues that light smokers face is they vary in their desire for nicotine. Some light smokers can feel the need to smoke once a day and then let it go. Others may find they can go for several days without the urge to smoke and then find themselves reaching for a smoke. Those who smoke in this way may tell themselves they aren't really smokers at all and can quit anytime they want. They also tend to underestimate the risks of smoking and the ease they might have in choosing to quit. This is why all those who smoke, vape, or use e-cigs in any amounts should stop smoking. If you are finding it hard to fully let go your overall addiction to nicotine and tobacco products, be aware that all kinds of help are available. Reaching out for assistance to permanently stop smoking will do much to help reduce the health risks you face each and every time you light up.

35. What over-the-counter methods are there to help me quit smoking?

Quitting smoking has a great many benefits. Once you make the decision not to smoke anymore, you'll be on the way to better health. As discussed earlier, some people can quit on their own without help. Only a tiny percentage of smokers can quit on their own and avoid smoking for the rest of their lives. Most people need assistance. There are many ways to get help to quit smoking. One of the most popular is with the use of over-the-counter methods. Items that are available over the counter are items that can be freely purchased if you are of certain age. This distinguishes them from items that can be purchased only with a prescription from a medical professional. Using over-the-counter methods to help with quitting can be useful. They can be taken anywhere at any time. Speak to a doctor if you're under eighteen in order to get permission to purchase them. Such methods have a good track record. They are only allowed on the market after undergoing extensive testing. For the smoker who is looking for a convenient way to begin the process of quitting, it's well worth exploring such possibilities. Each method has pros and cons. If one doesn't work, try another instead. The types of available over-the-counter methods include the nicotine patch, nicotine gum, and nicotine lozenges. Collectively these are known as nicotine replacement therapy. Many methods combine several forms of nicotine replacement at once. People might use the patch to provide them with a steady level of nicotine while using gum and lozenges to combat sudden cravings.

Nicotine Gum

Nicotine gum is a quitting smoking aid that does not require a prescription to use unless you're under eighteen. It's one of the commonly used methods to help control smoking cravings. It is portable and convenient. Users can stow it in a bag. Those who begin this method can use it as often as every hour. The gum requires a specific technique to release the nicotine inside. Bite off one section to activate it. Many people report that this taste is peppery and reminds them of spicy food. Once activated, the gum needs to be between the cheek and the gumline for users to get the maximum benefit. When people want more nicotine, they take another bite of the gum and bring it to the same place. This process can continue for up to half an hour before the gum has no more nicotine. The gum is often used in conjunction with other quitting methods. Using it in place of smoking drastically reduces exposure to many of the most dangerous chemicals found in cigarette smoke. It also means not exposing others to secondhand or thirdhand smoke. At the same time, using nicotine gum may not allow the user to fully wean off tobacco altogether. It can also cause lots of side effects. People might find that they need to use a lot of it just to get rid of those cravings. They are also exposing your mouth to nicotine, a substance that is known to be dangerous to the tissues inside. The use of nicotine gum can irritate the mouth and cause a range of problems such as stomach upset, jaw irritation, and excessive saliva production. For these reasons, experts suggest using this method only with great caution.

Nicotine Lozenges

As the name implies, these are small lozenges that people can suck on and get a dose of nicotine. Like nicotine gum, they use the nicotine lozenges as often as needed. The goal is to fend off cravings without smoking. The lozenges go between the cheek and gums. Suck on one and get nicotine. No need to go to a doctor to get access to the nicotine. They are available in several sizes. The mini lozenge version lets users get access to a quick dose of nicotine that can address cravings quickly. Unlike gum, people don't have to chew them. Sucking can help relieve oral cravings and help ward off the worst of the withdrawal effects. Given the small dose in the lozenge, the smoker may have to use a lot of them to satisfy cravings. Like nicotine gum, they can also irritate the mouth and give varied symptoms such as heartburn and nausea. Experts recommend using them in combination with other quitting methods and not using them longer than three months.

Nicotine Patches

The nicotine patch is a small patch of about two square inches on the skin. Originally available only by prescription, it has been an over-the-counter product since 1996. Many smokers have used them with great success. The patch has the benefit of being easy to use and not visible when worn under your clothing. People can quit smoking without the need to let others know they are a former smoker. There's no need to worry about the patch when it's on. Users can also pick from varied doses to find the one they like best. Research has shown this method has about double the rate of efficacy compared with attempting to quit cold turkey. Over time, the goal is to gradually reduce the dosage until they are able to overcome nicotine cravings. Users get a steady dose of nicotine as they wear it. Most people choose to keep the patch on between sixteen and twenty-four hours a day. It can also be used in combination with other methods. Keep in mind the patch is a good choice for those who are looking for something that's relatively easy. It can have some drawbacks. The amount of the nicotine the user is getting cannot be increased if they feel sudden cravings. Varied side effects have also been reported over the years. Many people choose not to wear it at night as it can disrupt sleep patterns. Some people feel nausea and other symptoms such as dizziness and headache. It's also important to remember that people should not smoke while wearing the patch as it can lead to a nicotine overdose. A typical former smoker will wear nicotine patches for eight to twelve weeks before quitting.

Nicotine Spray

Like the other methods mentioned, the nicotine spray can be used to ward off cravings. People will need a prescription for this one, but it can also help ward off sudden cravings. Put it under the tongue or inside the cheek. Many people find it easier to use than the gum. Sprays have the advantage in that they can be used when people like. They are convenient and handy. It can be used up to four times an hour. The spray brings the nicotine into the system relatively quickly. Some people find it a useful addition to their arsenal of quitting aids. Others find that it's not to their taste and prefer methods that are less bitter. Like other forms of smoking cessation, this one may cause side effects such as upset stomach. It's also best used in conjunction with other forms of quitting assistance such as counseling and support groups in order to see long-term success.

36. What kind of professional help is available?

Over-the-counter help with the process of quitting smoking can be of great use. These methods are easy to use and do not require the smoker to do more than buy something from a pharmacy if they are eighteen or older. While these methods are useful, many people find it even more helpful to combine them with other methods in order to fully wean themselves from smoking. Medical professionals can help smokers discover exactly which combination of methods might work best for you so they can completely stop smoking. The smoker might use an over-the-counter method in combination with counseling and assistance from medications as well as help via support groups and counseling sessions. The goal should be about quitting and finding methods that will bring about that long-term success.

Seven medications have been approved as of this writing to aid in efforts at quitting smoking. Three of them, the nicotine lozenge, nicotine gum, and nicotine patch, are available over the counter. Four more, the nicotine spray, inhaler, and two medications that don't have any nicotine, require a prescription for access. All smokers, including both social smokers and those who smoke a pack a day or more, can ultimately benefit. Talk to your parents or someone at school. They will help you decide if methods that need a prescription are right for you and how best to use them. Counseling, along with the use of medications, is a highly effective tool for a great many smokers.

As mentioned in the previous chapter, there are methods known as nicotine replacement therapy. While most such methods do not require a prescription, smokers will need a prescription for the nicotine nasal spray. The spray is delivered through the nostrils. It usually causes irritation during the first two days of use. Many people like it because it is easy to use and works rapidly. This method has also shown great promise for teens who are motivated to quit and looking for a convenient way to help get rid of a nicotine addiction. Users must make sure their hands are clean and the container is clean in order to avoid problems with contamination. It can be addictive, so it is best used with a combination of other methods.

In recent years, new medications have come on the market. These are meds that are designed to help reduce cravings. They do not put nicotine in the system, so they are often safer than some other methods as well as easier than quitting cold turkey. These medications help ward off cravings for tobacco. These medications are best used in conjunction with other forms of help such as counseling—a thoughtful plan to quit that takes into account the smoker's personal needs and lots of support from professionals and a peer group. The medications are known not to be habit forming, so users don't have to worry about getting addicted. Keep in mind these medications are generally only used for those who are eighteen and over. However, a doctor may advise people to consider them as they can help even if the smoker is under eighteen. Studies have shown them to be something that professionals should think about carefully when looking for the best ways to help teens become ex-smokers.

Zyban, also known as bupropion, is one of the most commonly used smoking cessation medications. It is taken in pill form. This medication is also widely prescribed for other medical conditions such as depression. Experts are not sure exactly how it helps combat such cravings, but they do know it can work really well when compared with other methods or a simple placebo. It should not be used under certain circumstances such as pregnancy or if the smoker has a history of other medical issues such as eating disorders and bipolar episodes. Users are instructed to create a plan that will get to them to nonsmoking state over a period of several weeks. They begin taking the medication a week before they plan to stop smoking. Most people take the medication once or twice a day with the goal of stopping within twelve weeks. Those who feel cravings for nicotine may use nicotine replacement therapy methods such as patches to help them function better during this period and cope with any withdrawal side effects. A doctor can help with close monitoring to help avoid any side effects and make sure this method produces the desired results.

Varenicline, or Chantix, is another medication commonly used to help smokers quit. It should only be taken if you are older than eighteen. Food and Drug Administration (FDA) officials specifically recommend against teens taking it at the present time. They do not believe it is effective in teens. If the smoker is of age to consider this medication, it is similar to Zyban. However, they will not be able to take it any form of nicotine replacement therapy. Like Zyban, users begin after making a plan to quit. A week before they plan to stop smoking, they'll start that first pill. Most people are able to tolerate it well with few reported side effects. It's easy to use and can double the chances of success in recommended age groups. While it can be a good way to overcome smoking urges and quit entirely, FDA officials have found that the medication can lead to very severe mood changes and even worsen an existing mental illness. It has also been linked to reports of suicidal ideation.

37. How can I tell my parents about my need to quit?

The decision to quit smoking is a monumental one. When teens decide to quit smoking, they are making a decision that will begin to pay off almost immediately. Kids who quit vastly decrease their chances of health problems compared to their peers who continue to smoke. If you want to take those first, tentative steps, one of the most important things you can do is seek out help and support from others. Parents provide the guidance teens need to decide how best to quit. They can offer the financial assistance the teen needs in order to pay for therapy and counseling. A parent who has quit smoking and continued to avoid smoking can help by offering their own personal experience and showing firsthand that quitting can be done. A parent can serve as the role model teens need to move past cravings and permanently bid goodbye to all forms of tobacco. A parent can also serve as a resource person if the smoker finds that quitting is really hard.

Letting parents know you smoke and then letting them know of your determination to quit can be a life-changing experience for you and an opportunity to let your parents be good parents at the same time. It's important to keep a few things in mind before you do anything else. You need to tell your parents the truth. Keep in mind your parents may already know that you smoke. It's not that hard to tell someone is smoking even just a few cigarettes here and there. Tobacco use leaves many telltale signs. Your parents may have noticed a distinct smell on your clothing after you've been in a room with other smokers. If you smoke at home, tobacco will leave a residue on the bedding and walls that can in turn give everything in the room an unnatural, brownish cast. After just a few short weeks of smoking, chances are it's obvious that you're short of breath and coughing more. Given these clues, most parents will at least suspect something's going on. That's the bad news. The good news is that telling your parents will open up doors of communication between you and your parents and set up the help you need in order to quit. If you've been thinking about telling your parents that you want to quit, it's a good idea to begin with a plan. Your goal is to help you both come to a place of understanding and then move forward from there.

You'll want to find a place and a time. A good place is a place where you both feel comfortable such as the basement or family room. A good time is when your parents have had some time to relax. This gives them the time to focus their full attention on you and what you're going to say. It can be helpful to rehearse before you begin. This gives you a sense of self-confidence before you start speaking. Your goal is to focus your parent's attention on the fact that you want to quit. If you have younger brothers and sisters, it's also best to speak when they are not around. Think about finding time when they're engaged in after-school activities or are asleep. It's also best to pick a private space. Telling your parents important news like this is best delivered in a private space away from crowds. This way, you'll know they hear what you have to say. You'll also know that no one else can listen on your private conversation. If you are worried about your parent's reaction, it can be useful to enlist someone at school. A counselor may be able to provide you with a private room at school where you can speak. They can also serve as your backup when you're in need of some support as you speak to them. The goal is to let them know what you're doing as well as your desire to quit. You might want to opt to speak to one parent rather than both at the same time. If you are closer to one parent, they can help you formulate a plan to let the other know what's going on in your life.

If one of your parents is a former smoker, they can provide you with the help you need to convince the parent who never smoked that you are sincere in wanting to quit. It's also best to do some research about methods that might help you quit. Presenting your parents with evidence of quitting methods provides additional evidence that you're planning to quit. Once you've picked a day and a time, you'll want to speak slowly and carefully. You might want to write up notes in advance to touch on as you speak to them. Ideally, you should let them know all about your smoking habit. Let them know approximately how many cigarettes you smoke in a given week. Tell them when you started to smoke and where you typically light up. If you've tried to quit on your own before, you should let them know that, too. Keep in mind that they might ask you about peers who smoke. That's a decision that you're better off leaving to your friends and their parents. Give your parents time to process this information. Even if they know that you smoke, it can be hard hearing it directly from you. Stay calm and listen to what they have to say in response. Think about handing them your cigarette stash or showing them where you keep it. This is a gesture of goodwill that indicates you are sincere about wanting to stop. You and your parents can then begin the process of finding you help and giving you that lifeline to leave cigarette smoking behind for good.

38. What effects might I experience once I begin quitting?

The decision to quit smoking or stop using e-cigs is quite a daring leap for many smokers. Many smokers don't make the choice in part because they are afraid what will happen to them once they start the process. Someone who uses e-cigs may want to quit but might not imagine it important. They worry that quitting will be hard and ultimately pointless. Smokers often think that since they've already damaged their bodies, it seems rather pointless to walk away. One of the most amazing things about quitting is just how quickly they'll start to feel better. In a few short days and weeks, they can put smoking behind them and carve out a whole new life. Before beginning, it's important to keep in mind that the smoker will most likely experience some symptoms. This is true for those who are using e-cigs as this form of nicotine will have similar effects. It is crucial to have a plan in place before they start. It's also hugely important to have a support system in place. Having support from friends and family means having people who can help the smoker get past those symptoms. Working with trained medical professionals can also offer the smoker the support they need to cope with any problems and find a solution that will help lessen the pain and ease their way forward. After quitting, people can expect many varying mental and physical effects. Not everyone will have the same experiences. Some people may have transient effects after they stop vaping that are over with quickly. Others may feel a wide variety of effects that can linger for some time. Most people find such symptoms will taper off within two weeks and completely disappear in a month. Such side effects may happen suddenly and then go away a short while later. Even if someone has been smoking or vaping only for a few weeks, they will probably have these problems once they've decided to let it go. Once they're done, they're done for good. They can look back on what they've done with a great sense of satisfaction. Most of the symptoms will peak between three and five days after they've stopped. This is the time when the smoker fully rids their body of nicotine, so it's especially important to have that support system in place and ready to help. It's also important to stay away from places where the smoker might be tempted to use e-cigs such as school bathrooms.

Many symptoms will have an emotional and physical component. Be prepared to feel cravings for tobacco and nicotine at unexpected times such as during class or at band practice. This is a perfectly normal feeling. Smokers may feel an overwhelming craving to light up. For most people, this will take over their feelings for a few minutes as often as once or twice an hour for an hour. These cravings happen, but they tend to last only a few minutes. Once the smoker is past those first few days, many smokers find they start to decrease in both frequency and intensity. Another common problem is having trouble sleeping. Sleep may be interrupted by sudden cravings before the smoker goes to sleep and once asleep. When not sleeping, the smoker might feel very restless. It can be hard to concentrate on other things when the smoker is concentrating on avoiding smoking. Speak with a counselor about techniques like deep breathing. These are ways to refocus attention on other things. It's very important to avoid caffeine. Once people quit smoking, they begin to absorb more caffeine. This can increase feelings of anxiety and restlessness and make it even harder to focus. Emotions can change quickly. People might get more annoyed with a younger brother or snap at a best friend unexpectedly. They might feel angry and annoyed or depressed and unwilling to leave home for after-school activities. These are common effects. This is why it is imperative to let people know of plans to quit smoking or vaping immediately. People who care about are those who want the smoker to succeed. They will be patient and understanding as the smoker works through this difficult process. Another thing to keep in mind is people often feel hungrier once they stop smoking or vaping. That's because smoking and vaping contain chemicals that can suppress appetite. Laying in healthy snacks before starting smoking-quitting attempts can help people pick better choices once they've stopped smoking. Keep favorite fruits and vegetables around the house. Bring them with you when traveling and at school. In addition to such feelings, people might notice physical problems that resemble a cold. Bouts of coughing and sneezing are common as well as sore throats that can make people feel frustrated and miserable. They might feel unexpectedly dizzy or lightheaded. They might also feel really tired. Many smokers have been relying on smoking and vaping to help them stay awake. When they stop, it's common to find they're falling asleep earlier at night and staying asleep longer. Constipation and headaches can also be a huge problem when ridding the system of nicotine. Common over-the-counter remedies can offer relief.

These symptoms can feel overwhelming at first. The best thing to do is understand what's happening and why. If the smoker can get through it for a few days, chances are they'll be able to walk away for good. When cravings begin, delay acting on them for a few minutes. This is usually enough to let the craving pass for a while. Get up and do something else. Drink water. Take a walk. Contact friends and ask for help. Remind yourself all the things that will get better once you're done with smoking. An ex-smoker saves money, has better endurance, and enjoys life. If you're a former smoker tempted to light up again, remind yourself this is not an excuse to quit. They'll only have to go through withdrawal symptoms again. If the first effort does not succeed, do not despair. You are not alone. It may take two, three, or even more tries to rid the body of nicotine addiction. Think about what didn't work the last time you tried to quit. Making new plans can help any smoker see what did not work and find out what will.

39. How can I help someone I care about quit?

Given how many risks smoking poses, it can be hard to see your parent, sibling, or close friend light up again and again. If you'd like to assist a loved one leave using cigarettes, e-cigs, or vaping behind forever, keep a few things in mind first. It's important to be supportive. It's also useful to provide them with accurate information and let them know how much you care. Helping someone you love quit is an act of profound respect and kindness. Even if it takes several attempts, you will have made a wonderful difference in their lives and the lives of everyone else around them along the way. Studies show about 70 percent of all smokers want to quit. The remainder may have spent time thinking about it and perhaps concluded it's too hard. In any year over a million people attempt to stop smoking and succeed. Over 40 percent of all smokers who have smoked since 1965 have permanently left smoking behind. With help, chances are your loved one can join them. Remember, quitting smoking can be one of the hardest things they'll ever do. You may have to deal with plenty of negative feelings and frustrations on their behalf while the quitting process is in process. It can take a few days to get nicotine from a person's system. It may take up to several weeks and even longer before your loved one has completed the entire journey. Your goal is to help them understand you are on their side and there for them.

If they haven't already made the decision to quit, gently ask them if they've thought about it. Many smokers are aware of the dangers of smoking. However, they might not be aware of all of the dangers it poses or why c-cigs and vaping can be just as dangerous. A smoker may be aware of the risk of lung cancer. They may not be aware of the risk of heart attack and stroke. They may not know that smoking, vaping, and using e-cigs can lead to vastly increased risks of additional cancers. A smoker may not know how smoking can lead to problems with sight or hearing as well as taste and touch. Your friend with asthma might not know just how much smoking or vaping can increase the frequency and severity of their attacks. A parent may be aware of such risks. They might not know about the reality of secondhand and thirdhand smoke. It's always a good idea to bring this to their attention. You can help your parent realize they may be harming not only their own health but your health and the health of your siblings as well. Remind them that secondhand smoking causes thousands of medical problems in others, including a vastly increased risk of lung cancer for you and your siblings. Even after bringing this up, remember it can take them some time to reach out and begin quitting. Planting the seeds now can help your loved one begin to realize that you're on their side and you care about them. It's a good idea to let them know that you have faith in their abilities. You believe they can quit. The choice to quit must be theirs. If they are not ready to take that first step, don't judge their decision. A smoker may decide to quit only to find it isn't working out. Each time they decide to quit, that's a good step. It's something they can learn from once they decide to make another attempt. Quitting tobacco and vaping is just as hard as quitting other drugs. You can help by helping them develop a plan to quit. Many people have developed routines in life that revolve around lighting up. Be there for your parents and friends when they might start smoking. If they are in the school bathroom with others who are vaping, help them walk away. Help a parent by making them a special breakfast for a few days that will shake up their routine and help them develop new, healthy habits. Let your best friend know they can talk to you about quitting. Be there to listen and cheer them up. Lay in a supply of items they can suck on instead. Sucking candies for smoking breaks and other times where vaping takes place is a good idea. Chop up vegetables for your parents or siblings, and put them in the fridge in easy reach. Help them settle into new routines. Ask parents for help with your homework. Plan outings after school and on weekends. A brisk walk or short bike trip can help them stave off cravings and help you bond at the same time. If you have friends who are smokers or who vape, avoid bringing them home or hanging out with them at school. With a parent's permission, take all smoking-related items and get rid of them. If your siblings or other close relatives smoke or vape, make sure they are avoiding your house right now. If they see a relative can quit, they might find the inspiration they need to quit. Now is the time to clean your house. Ridding it of all smoking stains and anything else from nicotine can help you and everyone in your family make a clean start. Do not take anything they say personally during this period. Withdrawal is hard. Be sympathetic as they attempt to rise past one of the toughest obstacles they'll ever face in life. You want them to succeed even if it takes a lot of time and effort. Once they have done it, throw them a big party. Quitting is a major achievement that deserves your every single second of applause.

40. What can I do to help others in my community who smoke?

Smoking isn't just a personal issue. It's a community concern. According to the CDC, illnesses from smoking and vaping impose billions of dollars in needless health-care costs. Such illnesses typically strike people in the prime of life, once they've completed their education and entered the workforce. Children are left without a father when a parent dies of a smoking-related heart attack. A child may develop cancer as a result of secondhand smoking or being exposed to vaping. Thirdhand smoking can coat any home's doors and other surfaces, triggering even more illness. Landlords need to spend hours scrubbing away dangerous chemicals that can be left behind by the trail of a single group of smokers. Smoking and vaping can lead to fires that can damage property and cost innocent lives. When smokers take smoking breaks outside, others are left to walk through smoke-filled outdoor spaces and pick up the slack at work when a smoker gets sick. The use of nicotine from vaping can lead to a loss of concentration, addiction, and money that would be far better spent elsewhere. These extra costs are over $20 every single day for every single smoker in the United States. That's a lot of lost money. It's also a lot of lost working hours and an even greater cost in human lives. Similar losses result from nicotine use via vaping and e-cigs. This is one of many reasons why communities all over the world have banded together to help combat this issue. Officials want to help people who smoke quit and help others avoid lighting up at all. If you've seen a loved one struggle with smoking, you know how hard it can be to quit. If you've tried to quit and finally succeeded, you know the allure smoking poses and how difficult it is to let go of this highly addictive substance. Knowing that, you may be wondering exactly what you can do to help others in your community who smoke and vape.

Start a Community or School Group

One of the best ways to help people who smoke and everyone around them is by starting a local community group. Contact local elected officials. They may already have a group that's all about antismoking efforts on a local level. Attending meetings can help people understand the specific challenges their peers and everyone else in the community face when it comes to combating the spread of smoking and vaping. Teens can do the same at school. Many schools allow students to begin a club focused on their interests. A club that is about assisting fellow students with smoking and vaping issues is a great way to really make a difference. Ask like-minded friends to join in. You and your friends can have a long-lasting impact on public health in your neighborhood. Antismoking education groups may even be eligible for funds to help begin the group and use it to reach out to others. Many teens know little, if anything, about the risks of vaping and e-cigs. You can change that.

Bring In Speakers

Ask for meeting spaces where people with a background in this subject can speak out. Many communities have spaces set aside for people to meet and talk. Those who have quit can tell everyone else how they did it. Health professionals can step up and share information about the dangers of smoking, e-cigs, and vaping. A good, honest, direct talk can have a huge impact on people's lives and create a lasting impression. Ask local officials if you can have time during a community meeting to bring attention to your efforts. A short presentation can create interest, generate excitement, and help publicize your activities to others. Ask teachers to give presentations during school pep rallies or during other events such as homecoming and the prom.

Hand Out Accurate Information

Create handouts filled with accurate information. Using graphics and bulletin points can open up lively dialogue and begin discussion. Think about your intended audience. Even kids in grade school can benefit from leaflets that explain why smoking is bad and how officials at e-cig makers deliberately target them. Hand out materials at schools as part of a club's activities. Distribute fliers at lunch and when everyone's heading home to attract attention. If you live in an apartment complex or a gated community, find out if you can get permission to hang fliers in common areas where people smoke and vape. Libraries are another place to hold meetings, get access to good sources of information, and speak out to others. A librarian can help with further information about the dangers of e-cigs and vaping.

Use Social Media

Social media is another way to get the antismoking and anti-e-cig message out. A social media page can offer basic information about community resources. This can also serve as a place to provide convenient updates about ongoing events and subjects of interest. If there is a local social media page, share this media page with them. Ask if you can post updates about your own group and plans. Reach out friends via social media to let them know about how to organize and respond to questions others might have. Post articles about smoking, vaping, and e-cigs.

Quitting Support Groups

Few things are harder than quitting smoking. Create a space where people going through the process can share their feelings and find support. Host the meeting at your house or as part of a school-based antitobacco and antivaping group. This should be a judgment-free space where everyone can find solace for their own personal journey. People can share their efforts at quitting. They can also share stories about helping others quit. A support group can also take place online. Letting people speak and leave anonymous comments can lead to greater exchanges of ideas and an increased sense of community.

41. What if I start smoking again?

Smoking has so many harmful effects. One of the most insidious is that it's very hard to quit. Quitting can be very easy. It's the remaining away from smoking and vaping that can be truly hard. Addiction to tobacco and nicotine gets into the brain and stays there. Nicotine will hijack your innate reward system. Once it does, those good feelings get tied up in wanting to get that reward system again and again. The brain makes associations that are very hard to shake. They think about something they enjoy, like a full brunch, and that feeling of enjoyment is tied into the cigarette they smoke with it or the e-cig they use afterward. Under those circumstances, it's hardly surprising that it might take more than one attempt at quitting. Relapses are common. They are not a moral failing or an indication that the person can't stop smoking. A smoker might have sworn off cigarettes for good. Then, one day, friends start to light up or offer an e-cig pod. All of a sudden, the smoker is grabbing a smoke or vaping with them. They might not be smoking a pack again, but they're definitely bumming a few smokes and some vapes a few times a week. When this happens, the smoker is not alone. A study in the June 2014 issue of *Addictive Behaviors* looked at smokers over twenty years. The study found that nearly 40 percent had a relapse during that time frame. The good news is that almost 70 percent were able to get past the relapse and stop smoking going forward. All smokers can do the same. It's important to recognize and understand why someone might choose to start smoking again.

Triggers can be all around the smoker. Users see friends smoking or vaping and start to think it's unfair they can smoke but they can't. They also then start to feel deprived and maybe even angry. Even a single image of someone smoking and vaping or being around someone smoking or having brief company around a current smoker can set in place a series of events that the former smoker may not consciously realize. A smoker might find they are thinking about that cigarette or the e-cig pod for days or even weeks afterward. As they do, they can fall into a pattern of thought that's not productive. Feeling that someone is being deprived by not smoking or vaping anymore is not healthy. The smoker might still be thinking that smoking or vaping has some inherent value in life. When people see someone smoking, they start to think that person is being allowed to enjoy life while they're deliberately being deprived of pleasures. As they continue to feel that way, they're setting up their eventual return to smoking or vaping again. After the smoker has stopped smoking for some time, it's easy to think about those days as a smoker or vaper with a certain sense of nostalgia. As physical symptoms start to clear up, it can be very hard to remember all that lousy stuff that went with it. When the smoker is no longer coughing or struggling to climb up a set of stairs, those can seem like long ago days with little relevance today. All the really lousy stuff can seem of little importance when compared with the feel of a smoke in your hand as you watch your friends take long and happy puffs or enjoy a hit from an e-cig pod. Even after someone is no longer smoking and the nicotine is out of their system, the habit of having the smoke or the e-cig in the hands still lingers in the mind and can still influence how the person thinks and feels even when they are not expecting it. The simple act of sitting outside on a favorite park bench can recall when a person sat there smoking or vaping. Smoking and using e-cigs can be intimately intertwined with life experiences and personal habits. Short of moving away, there are many things the ex-smoker can do when they feel that habit again. People can break free of the hold of tobacco and nicotine again even when they're back to smoking. Millions of people have been down this path before and have found further success.

An ex-smoker may be tempted to use this time to simply continue to smoking again and become a smoker, but remember you have it in you to stop again. Now is the time to have a look at the reasons the smoker stopped and how they managed to find a way out. Take some time to remember what it was like to get out of breath and have stained clothing. Try recalling all the most unpleasant aspects of the time as a smoker. Think about the route taken last when it came to quitting then. If you have a list of prior reasons for stopping, you might still have it on hand now. Get it out, and start adding to it. Keep that list whenever you feel the urge to light up again. Have a look at all the bad things that smoking and using e-cigs will do to the body and mind. Reread the answers in this book for a reminder of exactly how smoking can ruin your life and your health. Now is also the time to seek out support again. You can find it online and in person. A single smoke doesn't mean you have to embrace smoking again. It's also the time to remember to take it on a daily basis. You've resisted the urge to smoke for so long. You can do it again and again. All you need is a single day, and then you can add to those days and quit smoking the same way you did before. Take inspiration knowing that you did the hard part of quitting once before and you can do it again. Like so many others, just because you've gone back to smoking again doesn't mean you can't go back to quitting again. The key is not to let that relapse redefine yourself as a smoker in the future. You were an ex-smoker. You can become an ex-smoker again. Be patient. Do not think of yourself as a smoker. You are someone who can become a former smoker and continue to remain one forever.

42. Is quitting smoking harder than quitting drinking?

Teens who smoke are also likely to drink alcohol. In every state in the union, only those twenty-one and over are legally allowed to purchase alcohol. This doesn't stop kids from getting access to alcohol. They might have a drink now and then at a party or sneak a drink from mom and dad's stash. Alcohol use is quite common across the country. It's more common than smoking and generally more socially accepted. There's a vast difference between alcohol and tobacco consumption. According to the Mayo Clinic, moderate, legal adult alcohol consumption may actually have certain benefits. In the past, when it was very hard to purify water, people of all ages largely drank watered-down alcohol for hydration. Today, we know that women who have up to one drink a day and men who have up to two may be protected from heart disease, stroke, and even diabetes. At the same time, studies also indicate that alcohol may be a factor in the development of certain cancers. Drinking and driving can lead to serious consequences. Over time, consumption of excessive amounts of alcohol may cause problems. Studies indicate that about eighteen million Americans struggle with addiction to alcohol in the United States. That's roughly one in twelve people. Like smoking, addiction to alcohol is often formed at home and at school. A parent or peer may share their love of drinking at the same time they introduce someone to using cigarettes, chewing tobacco, or vaping. Over time, the teen might find they have issues with alcohol and tobacco use. For those who are planning to quit, the question may become which of the two negative addictive behaviors they might wish to address first. For many people, the two are linked. They have a drink as they vape or smoke at a party. The urge to have a drink may trigger the urge to smoke, or they might light up and then reach for the whiskey sour. There is a link between smoking and drinking. Studies by the National Institute on Alcohol Abuse and Alcoholism have found that about 40 percent of all adult drinkers are also adult smokers. Only about 15 percent of people who have never smoked have indicated they are drinkers.

Alcohol and nicotine addiction have lots of factors in common. Research has suggested that drinking increases the pleasures of smoking. The same is true of smoking. Smoking and drinking at the same time may act in tandem, increasing the chances that a smoker will drink and vice versa. Alcohol and tobacco work on the same areas of the brain, providing users with many similar feelings. People smoke or vape, and the tobacco gets into their brains rapidly. This leads to a rush of pleasurable sensations for the smoker. Over time, this feeling fades. Smokers may go a long time between one cigarette and the temptation to use it again. A similar process is at work when drinking alcohol. When people drink, the brain releases chemicals that light up the pleasure centers of the brain. Like tobacco and nicotine, these feelings are temporary. Once the alcohol has left the body, the smoker is left wanting more. Tobacco and nicotine use differ from the use of alcohol because, as shown in previous chapters, there is no safe level of smoking. Even a single cigarette can lead to all sorts of increased health risks. Light to moderate alcohol does not carry the same overall health problems. However, heavy drinking can lead to health issues including the risk of many types of cancers. For those who are confronting both an addiction to smoking and an addiction to alcohol, the question may be where to begin.

People who smoke and drink may claim that the decision to continue smoking makes it easier for them to follow through on the process of getting past alcohol addiction. Researchers at Yale University looked into this claim. According to a paper submitted to the *Proceedings of the National Academy of Sciences*, the researchers found that smoking actually led to increased cravings for alcohol, making it harder for the smokers to complete alcohol addiction treatment programs. Another study from Yale found that "smokers who drink heavily have a tougher time quitting cigarettes than smokers who drink moderately or not at all." The two behaviors can go hand in hand, making it harder to quit either one. Those who smoke and drink also up their risks for all kinds of health issues. Quitting smoking and quitting tobacco use also share similar processes. Like quitting tobacco and nicotine, walking away from alcohol use may take repeated tries. The alcoholic may need help from multiple sources in order to finally manage the process of quitting for good. Each addiction may lead to failed attempts and can take time to complete. Those who have quit using alcohol may find it easier to quit smoking once they decide it's time. This is because the process of quitting smoking and the process of stopping alcohol use often require a similar ability to decide to stop doing something and the determination to see it through. Similar principles can apply to quitting smoking that mark the process of quitting alcohol use. A smoker will often find it helpful to find a support group. The physical process of withdrawing from nicotine use versus the process of withdrawing from alcohol use, however, may differ. Long-term drinkers may have far more intense symptoms, including tremors and hallucinations, that are not seen when people stop using tobacco. Nicotine affects fewer neurotransmitters in the brain than alcohol does. Once the initial stage of washing alcohol and tobacco out of the body has passed, the remaining steps toward ceasing smoking and ceasing alcohol use have much in common. The two processes make use of steps that have been shown to work. Quitting smoking is always the right choice. Anyone who drinks more than moderate levels as defined by health officials should also explore avenues of quitting. Leaving smoking and drinking behind will improve your overall health and make it easier for you to be around for the people you love.

43. What kinds of new treatments are being developed to help people quit?

Medicine never stands still. New ways of doing things are always on the horizon. Doctors want to serve their patients better and help them find pathways to health. When it first became officially clear in the 1960s that tobacco use was dangerous, doctors, health officials worldwide, and scientists began to search for ways to help their patients stop smoking. This process is ever changing and evolving today. Research about how best to help people quit smoking continues in studies and laboratories all over the world. If something doesn't work for them, there are many different possible treatments that just might. One thing to bear in mind is that vaping will not help you quit. According to the experts at Johns Hopkins, "Although they've been marketed as an aid to help you quit smoking, e-cigarettes have not received Food and Drug Administration approval as smoking cessation devices. A recent study found that most people who intended to use e-cigarettes to kick the nicotine habit ended up continuing to smoke both traditional and e-cigarettes."

Antinicotine Vaccines

One of the most promising of all antismoking treatments currently under investigation is an antinicotine vaccine. The idea behind the antinicotine vaccine is simple. Scientists want to figure out ways to bring the immune system to attack nicotine molecules before they reach your brain. This should prevent smokers from craving nicotine and getting rid of the desire to smoke. Initial trials were promising but were not brought to market. That's because they were only effective in about 30 percent of participants. Researchers are working on different formulas in an effort to better improve the efficacy of the vaccine. A new formula that focuses on a quality known as handedness, which refers to how molecules fit, is being aimed at the fact that the most common form of nicotine is a left-handed molecule. Using this strategy created a vaccine that was 60 percent effective in mice. Scientists are hopeful that this avenue of attack may one day lead to a vaccine or a series of fast vaccines that can induce the body to let go of nicotine addiction for good. They believe this may also one day apply to other kinds of addictive substances including alcohol, heroin, and cocaine.

Sex-Based Differences

Another area of research has been into the differences between quitting patterns in men and women. Women smoke in lower numbers than men.

However, women may face special challenges when quitting. Researchers at Yale who study smokers have found that women are more vulnerable than men to the complications of smoking. They report that "studies have shown that women are more susceptible to tobacco-related health conditions such as cardiovascular disease, respiratory disease, and stroke. Women who smoke also experience increased risks of cervical cancer, lower bone density, estrogen deficiency disorders, menstrual cycle disorders, conception delay, infertility, and pregnancy complications. Since 1987, lung cancer has surpassed breast cancer as the number one cause of cancer death for women." Research has also shown that some smoking-quitting methods may not work as well for women. The nicotine patch, for example, does not appear to work as well for women who are trying to quit. Researchers have learned that women smoke for different reasons than men. Women often use smoking to help control their weight. Women may be less motivated to remain an ex-smoker if smoking leads them to gain weight. They are also more likely to smoke again after a relapse. Certain medications such as varenicline may act more quickly in women, giving the head start they need to keep away from smoking for good.

Smart Technology

Technology is another area that can be used to harness help people quit. Many different apps on the market can offer detailed help. Some charge a nominal fee, and others are free. The National Cancer Institute has an app specially designed to help you with your quitting journey. The app has many useful features. Users get access to a quitting date, reminders how much they're saving once they quit, and help such as a text messaging service that gives them backup any time of the day. Other apps have additional features that can give any smoker that extra backup whenever they need it. The MyQuit Coach app has been approved by physicians. Users can pick their quitting options and get access to a community of like-minded people. Cessation Nation is another free app with help like fun games to take your mind off of wanting a cigarette. SmokeFree is a free app that's like having a friend along for the ride. The use of such smart technology allows people to access help from anywhere at any time.

Other Areas of Promise

One of the goals of modern medical practice is to seek out new ways to account for individual differences in physiology. Each person is different. Researchers are trying to examine new ways to make these differences work for each person. Some people may metabolize nicotine more quickly than others. They may be more at risk of getting hooked on tobacco and finding it harder to quit. Precision medicine can help identify individuals with this predisposition and then give them medications and therapy designed for their genetic profile. Behavioral modification is another area of ongoing research. Studies indicate smokers need not always come in to an office for counseling. Telephone counseling has proven highly effective. Having a counselor make follow-up calls can be especially effective by providing smokers with someone they can trust. Investigators are exploring emotional and mental help in antismoking assistance. Cognitive behavioral therapy can be used along with medications to help smokers identify triggers and help them find coping behavior that can ward off cravings for good. Researchers are also examining the ideal way to help teens quit. Teens need special care when trying to quit. A combination of varied methods including making use of primary pediatric care settings as well as behavioral assistance has shown a great deal of promise.

44. How can I become part of the antismoking and antivaping movement?

For a long time, tobacco and nicotine product was quite common. A significant percentage of Americans smoked. Since that time, efforts have helped reduce the number of American smokers drastically. Only about one in twenty teens smoke. This came about because of many factors including the hard work of brave professionals who have helped save countless lives. It's not only professionals who have made a difference. Grassroots efforts have been in place for decades. Today, while fewer teens are smoking, many more are using nicotine products in the form of vaping and e-cigs. Much remains to be done to help reduce such numbers and help people quit for good. A teen reading up this subject may be wondering what steps they can personally take to get more involved and become a peer leader.

One way to engage with others is to look for help from outside sources that have been engaged in long-standing efforts to fight against the dangers of tobacco and nicotine use. Organizations such as the American Heart Association, American Cancer Society, and American Lung Association all have sections that are devoted specifically to the dangers of smoking. Contacting such organizations directly as well as online can provide a wealth of resources filled with accurate antismoking and antivaping information. The CDC has a Youth Tobacco Prevention page that can help teens find additional information and resources for everything related to teen nicotine and tobacco use.

Many organizations are aimed specifically at teens. For example, Truth Initiative aims to inspire people to lead lives free of tobacco. Officials here "give young people the facts about tobacco and the industry behind it, engage individuals and groups to make change in their communities, innovate ways to end tobacco use and join forces with collaborators committed to a tobacco-free future." Other organizations offer equally useful support. The Campaign for Tobacco-Free Kids organizes many varied efforts designed to discourage teen tobacco use, both in the United States and across the globe. Teens can join in their efforts to learn more about the dangers of smoking, talk to peer groups, and make it easier to avoid exposure to tobacco and nicotine products. Students Working against Tobacco has offices in several states, including Florida and Oklahoma. The Youth Engagement Alliance for Tobacco Control aims to help strengthen efforts by teens to combat tobacco use in their communities. Student leaders can learn about the dangers of smoking and vaping and how best to convey this information to their peers.

❖

Case Studies

1. MONIQUE IS A TEENAGE SMOKER AND VAPER

Monique is sixteen and a half. She's headed into her junior year of high school. She's spent a lot of time thinking about what she wants to do once she graduates. Her interests include music, math, and cooking meals with recipes that have been handed down from her circle of extended family members. She's seriously thinking about entering culinary school in a few years and making her passion for food her life's work. She has a few close girlfriends whom she likes to hang out with on weekends and sometimes after school. The large urban high school she has been attending since ninth grade is one of the better schools in her area. It's a long commute. She has to take a bus and two separate trains to get there. She likes how it feels when she enters the doors. Her teachers are enthusiastic and caring. There are a number of classes not available in her district high school. She's been taking formal cooking lessons. There are no metal detectors to get inside or lingering areas of graffiti understaffed school custodians have yet to remove. While the school is a good fit, she finds the trip means an early morning and getting home later than some of her peers. As a night owl, it can be tough for her to get up and run out. She's only one of a handful of students in her area who've ventured so far away from home. Sometimes she gets lonely and wonders if it's all worth it just to go to school. She doesn't tell her friends, but she's proud she's stuck with it. She gets good grades and fits in with her peers at school and at home.

About a year and a half ago after she first started school, Monique felt a sense of anxiety. She had a school counselor she liked and was starting to make friends. She was pleased at herself for taking a risk and going to a new school in a new part of town. Still, something was missing. After an invite to attend a free concert at a park not too far from the new school, she found herself with a group of friends from school and their stash of standard cigarettes along with a vaping machine. Monique's mom told her not to smoke, and so did a few of her cousins. Another relative told her she'd tried to quit a few times and found it really hard going before she was finally able to stop. She ignored her friends' suggestions to try it for about half an hour. Wanting to fit in and noticing that everyone else was doing the same thing, she took her first cigarette. After the first few puffs, she started to cough violently. Her friend told her it would stop after a few more inhalations. She really wanted to stop, but she was afraid of looking out of place and becoming a teacher or parent in scold mode. The last thing she wanted to do was make her friends feel bad. People also passed around the vaping mechanism. She tried dipping. The liquid drops hit the coil, and then she inhaled the vapor. She felt fine afterward. After a few days, she began to feel a craving for more nicotine. She had some pocket money from a few babysitting jobs. She wanted to put it away to help her with her culinary school plans. Lately, she's been spending more and more of her money on cigarettes. She's also bought a vaping machine and stowed it where she thinks her mom and little sister can't find it. She's really worried that she'll be discovered, but she feels like she needs a few e-cig pods a week to help her cope with the hours she spends away from home. She puts them in a separate bag and keeps them in her locker. On weekends, she vapes with a friend who also goes to her school and lives in her neighborhood. The friend's mom doesn't think vaping can hurt, so she lets her daughter and guests do it outside or in the basement.

Analysis

Like many smokers and vapers, Monique first began smoking when she was still in her teens. Almost 90 percent of all smokers begin smoking before they turn nineteen. Many start to smoke because they have peers who are doing the very same thing. They find themselves in the midst of a social group where they want to fit in. Smoking and vaping offer an easy way for teens to show they are not afraid to go against the prevailing wisdom and do what a mom or teacher might warn against. Smoking and vaping can also be a means of coping with the stress of a new place. Monique's first experience of smoking is a common one for many teens.

She may not like it initially, but she does it to fit in. Her use of vaping is also very typical. E-cigs are the most widely used form of tobacco in the United States in the nineteen and under peer group. Like her peers, Monique doesn't think vaping is harmful. The adult who lets her smoke is also typical in her belief that using e-cigs is not a dangerous thing to do. About 25 percent of Monique's peers choose to engage in dripping as they believe it will produce a more intense vapor and better flavor. Her use of cigarettes and vaping at the same time is also very common. Studies indicate teens were more likely to indicate they smoked if they were also using e-cigs. Vaping can act as a gateway for further and even more damaging use of tobacco and nicotine products. Despite the prevalent belief that the two are not linked, e-cigs can make using cigarettes more socially acceptable. Teens who use e-cigs are also less likely to quit smoking. Neither parents nor teens should assume using e-cigs is a harmless practice. Teens should also avoid using both cigarettes and e-cigs as both can lead to lifelong health issues.

2. ETHAN IS CONCERNED ABOUT HIS BOYFRIEND'S SMOKING

Ethan is a nineteen-year-old college freshman. He was admitted to the pre-vet program at a highly regarded state university. His boyfriend is attending a nearby college. The boyfriend is majoring in education with the goal of becoming a high school English teacher. This is the first time Ethan has been away from home for such a long time to study. He's a bit overwhelmed with the amount of studying he needs to do just to keep up with the work required for his prestigious program. He wants to get the best grades possible so that he can get into an esteemed grad program and do further research in veterinary studies. Part of his coursework has been studying advanced biology classes under the close supervision of an advisor. His advisor is an ex-smoker and ardent antismoking activist.

Ethan's boyfriend has been smoking and vaping for several years. While Ethan has been aware of the possible negative effects of smoking, it's only in the last few months that his eyes have truly been opened to the dangers his boyfriend faces as he continues to smoke and vape. Ethan's dorm and many other areas of the campus prohibit smoking and vaping. Smoking is also not allowed within thirty feet of all building entrances. This makes it hard for them to meet on campus for dates. Similar policies exist at his boyfriend's dorm, so the boyfriend has been vaping more than he has in the past as it is far less noticeable. Ethan's boyfriend has attempted to quit several times in the past. Each time, despite support from Ethan and from known quitting aids, his boyfriend has been unable to overcome his urge to smoke and vape. Ethan is getting more and more worried that his boyfriend is going to face terrible health consequences as he grows up. Already he's noticed that his boyfriend seems to have physical problems. His friend is coughing more and seems to have less and less stamina. No matter what they're doing, Ethan has noticed that his friend always seems to be reaching for a new cigarette or e-cig more often than ever before. He's also noticed that his boyfriend doesn't seem as interested in being active. They used to like to do things together, like take hikes and go swimming. He was chalking up his boyfriend's issues to the changes they've both faced in their new setting. More than ever, he's convinced that he needs to do all he can to get his boyfriend to quit for good. He's not sure where to begin. Ethan's boyfriend has attempted to quit in the past, but it didn't stick. As Ethan spends more and more time immersed in his scientific studies, he's learned how to read scientific studies firsthand. Doing so has convinced him that he needs to find a way to help his boyfriend quit permanently. At the same time, he's afraid of creating friction in his relationship. He's worried that his boyfriend will get upset if he brings up the subject. He knows his boyfriend knows the dangers of cigarettes and e-cigs. His boyfriend has already tried to quit several times and has not been successful. He doesn't want to be a nag. He just wants to help someone he loves live a longer, better, healthier life.

Analysis

Ethan's dilemma is a common one. About 15 percent of Americans smoke. Only about 5 percent of teens smoke. However, many more are vaping. Many teens who vape also smoke. Many smokers would like to quit. They've tried and failed repeatedly. Helping a loved one stop smoking can be a difficult task. A young person may not be aware of the dangers of smoking. They might not know about the dangers of smoking or assume they are far in the future. As Ethan learns about the dangers smoking poses, it's not surprising that he's becoming more and more concerned about his friend's health. The fact that Ethan's boyfriend has tried to quit several times indicates he's also aware of such dangers. Ethan is trying to find a way to convince his boyfriend to make that choice stick. The fact that his dorm and much of the campus are smoke-free zones can serve as his ally. Ethan's boyfriend is unable to smoke when he's visiting. His boyfriend's reliance on e-cigs indicates that the boyfriend is aware of the need to be careful of such strictures. Ethan can make a concerted effort to help his boyfriend by providing him with more evidence about the negative effects of this product. He can also help his boyfriend by being as supportive as possible during the process of quitting. Helping his boyfriend can serve as a means of bonding between the two of them and ultimately strengthen their relationship. People who have someone they can count on as they quit are those who are more likely to navigate the process successfully.

3. NICOTINE IS AFFECTING LUCIANA'S ATHLETIC PERFORMANCE

For as long as she can remember, Luciana has been a runner. Her mom talks with great affection about her toddler daughter's first steps. She loves to recount how Luciana's chubby little legs went from walking to running in about two hours. Luciana runs just about every single day. The early morning hours when she heads to school to get in some training are the best of her week. She's a high schooler immersed in her high school's team sports. She's the captain of the girl's track team and loves to urge her teammates to strive for greatness with each practice. Her personal specialty is the four hundred meters. It gives her time to think about the race as it unfolds. There's time for strategy and pacing. When she's not running track, the seventeen-year-old high school senior is heavily involved in other school sports. She's a member of the school tennis team and an alternate on the badminton squad. Her hand-eye coordination and ability to head down the courts really fast have rapidly made her a school favorite for local fans. In between her athletics, Luciana studies carefully. She has a solid B+ average in some very challenging classes. Her SAT scores were also very good. She hopes to become the first generation of her family to go to college. With her impressive results on the field, she's already getting attention from coaches and hints that scholarship offers could be on the way very soon. Luciana has been thinking about majoring in political science. She wants to return home and run for office day with the aim of really making a difference in her local community.

One day, Luciana was a little tired. She'd been running for hours, and it probably showed on her face. A fellow athlete introduced her to the use of nicotine. The friend compared it to a cup of coffee as a stimulant that was safe and wouldn't hurt her. She thought it was very safe compared to smoking. That was two years ago. Since then, she's been using nicotine in the form of vaping and other kinds of nicotine like chewing tobacco. Several of her teammates do the same. Her coach has noticed it, but she hasn't said anything as she did the same when she was a top runner at the national championships. Sometimes Luciana believes it helps her. She feels a sense of adrenaline and alertness when she's training. It isn't banned at sports meets, so she brings some with her when she's traveling. At home, she's less reliant on it. She thinks that her parents know about her use and don't approve of her use. She has five younger siblings. She's worried that they'll find her store of nicotine-related products and out her use even more to others in the community. She's also worried that they might tell her parents before she's ready to bring it up. She's also concerned about possible long-term effects. Sometimes, it feels as if the nicotine is helping. Lately, though, she's starting to feel that the use of nicotine products is hindering her sports performance rather than helping it. She wants to break free from it for good, but she's not sure where to begin. She knows the National Collegiate Athletic Association (NCAA) has banned the use of nicotine, so she needs to quit before she heads for college.

Analysis

Luciana is not alone in her use of nicotine products. Studies indicate about half of all athletes use nicotine in some form. The number of athletes who use nicotine is on the rise. Many athletes are exposed to nicotine products when part of a team. Professional athletes have often been seen using many kinds of nicotine and tobacco products. Athletes believe that it can help improve their concentration, keep body weight down, and provide both a sense of relaxation and a surge of energy as needed for high-stakes meets. An athlete can find nicotine products in many forms such as e-cigs and nicotine gum that are easy to conceal from others. Nicotine is banned by NCAA, but it is not banned by the Olympics or many local athletic organizations. Coaches tend to liken it to the use of caffeine, seeing it as a drug that does not need a lot of attention or concern. There is a need to educate many athletes, coaches, and others involved in athletics about the dangers the substance poses. Athletes should be encouraged to avoid starting smoking at all. They should also be heavily cautioned against the use of products like e-cigs, vaping, and other items that may contain this substance. In the long term, the use of nicotine products will have detrimental effects on the performance and health of any athlete who uses such products. Luciana and her teammates should be given access to resources that can help them stop.

4. TYLER WANTS TO HELP HIS PARENTS QUIT

Tyler is a freshman at a local community college. He took a year off after graduation to travel and think about his next steps. He didn't find his academic focus until after he left high school. Community college offered a low-cost alternative that would let him begin to explore possibilities. He really likes the idea of becoming a lawyer. In the meantime, he's decided on a concentration in paralegal studies. This will let him earn some money and get some practical experience before applying to law school. As an only child, he's been the center of attention at home since birth. Both his parents were older than the parents of his peers when he was born. They have a blue-collar background. His mom has a GED, while his dad never completed high school. His mom is a teacher's aide and his dad a truck driver. He respects their hard work and appreciates all they've done to provide him with a nice home.

He has lots of aunts and uncles. Two years ago, his aunt Mary developed emphysema. She was once a vibrant woman who loved nothing more than to spend time with him and invite him for big family dinners with his cousins. In the last year, he's noticed how pale and worn she looks. She spends most of her time on the couch at home hooked to an oxygen machine. Her prognosis is grim. He's becoming increasingly concerned with own parents. They're also heavy smokers. They smoke everywhere in the house including outside. His mom also smokes in his room as she tidies up. His dad likes to smoke with his buddies when he's playing poker and in the morning before heading out for work. His dad has a constant cough but so far no evidence of any other health problems. His mom doesn't seem as affected yet, but he would like her to quit. She doesn't smoke at work, but she smokes on weekends and when she's out with her close friends. Tyler doesn't smoke. He tried it once, but his friends prefer to use e-cigs rather than smoking. E-cigs look like children's toys to him, so they are not something he wants to try. When he was touring Europe, he saw smokers everywhere and quickly came to hate the smell. Tyler is very excited about the prospect of returning to his studies. But he's really worried about his parents. They're getting older. He wants his parents to be there when he gets into law school, graduates, and starts his own prac- tice devoted to international law. Tyler knows that smoking can be hard to quit. His aunt told him all about her struggles. She also told him that she begged her brother to stop smoking, but he told it was too hard. Tyler wants to gently push his parents to stop smoking. He's worried that if he does, they'll just push him away. He knows that his parents also drink and would like to help them cut down on drinking at the same time.

Analysis

Watching a loved one engage in counterproductive behaviors can be painful. Many teens are well aware of the dangers of smoking. A par- ent may know that smoking is not good for their health. They may not know just how much smoking can harm them. Older people often grew up in communities where smoking was part of the social scene. Tyler sees his parents smoking and feels helpless. He knows smoking is a terrible thing for them to do, but he's not sure where to begin to reach out to them. Tyler's parents also drink alcohol to excess. This is a common trait among those who smoke. Many alcoholics believe that quitting smoking and quitting drinking are too hard for them to do at the same time. They may never start the process of quitting at all. Another issue that many older smokers do not understand well is how their smoking can impact others. Research has continued to reveal the dangers of both secondhand and thirdhand smoking. Thirdhand smoking is a particularly new concept that is still being investigated. A smoker may not be aware of the trail of smoke they leave as they smoke. They also may not know about how this harms Tyler. She's also probably not aware that smoking can create issues in their entire home such as off-gassing from thirdhand smoke. Tyler has many options when speaking to his parents. He can start by speaking to his counselors at school. They have lots of material about helping smokers quit. He should speak to them directly and offer them varied kinds of support methods. He can also help them reduce their level of alcohol consumption by quitting smoking. Tyler lives at home. Pointing out their smoking is putting him in danger has been shown to help parents quit. Parents who are alerted to the problems smoking poses for their children are more likely to stop smoking. With his help and accurate information, Tyler can be the resource person his parents need.

5. RACHEL WANTS TO REDUCE HER RISK OF CANCER

Rachel is eighteen. If she could pick one word to describe herself, it would be "social." She's a bubbly person with hundreds of friends. At her high school, she's the center of attention. Her warm personality and welcoming ways have made her a favorite friend. She's been a resident of the same small suburban town since her parents moved here when she was three. She's gone from grade school to junior high school and high school with a large group of people. They're a close-knit bunch. As she thinks about college, she's also thinking about other things. Rachel has lots of interests. She's an excellent artist with a quick eye for detail. She also loves to read and write novels in her spare time. At school, she's been part of many activities including the second lead in the school play, the glee club, and raising money for a local animal shelter. She's planning to attend her state school and perhaps major in art history, French, or plant biology. She's really excited about her future. Her boyfriend is also going to college with her next year. They're already talking about getting married and starting a family once they've both graduated.

While she's a very optimistic person, one of the few things she worries about is her family history. Her grandmother died of breast cancer. She has several cousins who've been diagnosed with ovarian cancer. Her own mom had a mastectomy a few years ago. She's doing fine now, but Rachel worries her mom might have another bout of cancer. She's the oldest of three sisters. She hasn't been tested for any kind of personal cancer risk, but she realizes there's a pattern there and makes her think about her own future. She hasn't spoken to a doctor yet. Rachel smokes a little now and then. She also vapes. In her large circle of friends, this is a very common behavior. When she goes to the bathroom, she sees a lot of kids vaping. She isn't a heavy smoker like some of her friends. If you asked her, she'd say she was a social smoker. Rachel consumes a handful of cigarettes each week and a few rounds of vaping. She doesn't crave it very often. She mostly does it on weekends around her friends. With all the cancer in her family, she's started to become more and more concerned about her personal risks. The breast cancer has taken a toll on her mom. She recently looked up her background on a common website devoted to exploring ancestral links. She found out that reproductive cancers have stalked her family for generations. Rachel would like to stop smoking and vaping. She's troubled at the thought that she could be triggering her own risk of cancer. She's also disturbed at the possibility that she might be setting a bad example for her younger sisters. They know that she vapes and smokes. She doesn't want to make it seem like a normal activity.

Analysis

Cancer is a universal condition. About one-third to one-half of all Americans will get cancer at some point in life. With so many relatives with a cancer diagnosis, Rachel probably faces an above-average risk compared to the rest of the population. She may want to get more testing in order to indicate her exact risk. Her concern about smoking increasing her chances of getting cancer is understandable. Smoking increases the smoker's risks of just about every type of cancer. Smokers are at far more risk from everything from skin cancer to pancreatic cancer. If no one smoked, lung cancer would be a rare disease instead of one that kills thousands of Americans annually. Smoking has also been indicted in reproductive cancers. Studies have repeatedly linked smoking with many types of reproductive cancers, including ovarian and breast cancers. The nicotine found in vaping can lead to cell damage that triggers cancer. Rachel doesn't smoke or vape that often. As a so-called social smoker, she may think that her health risks are lower than heavier users. As pointed out in previous chapters, even light vaping and cigarette use can drastically increase the user's risk of cancer. Rachel should look for help to wean herself from vaping and cigarette use entirely. Products such as nicotine replacement therapy and school counseling can help her with this process. Once she makes the decision to quit, over time her risks of cancers will fall dramatically and continue to decrease. She should consider speaking with her peers about a group effort to quit smoking and vaping together. Creating a support group of friends devoted to the same goal can help all involved permanently stop smoking and vaping.

Glossary

Addiction: Addiction is a condition that is defined by the inability to consistently abstain from using a certain substance. This condition often involves efforts to stop using a certain substance that make take many efforts to be successful. Treatment can help tobacco and nicotine users overcome their addiction and successfully quit.

Centers for Disease Control and Prevention: Founded in 1946, the Centers for Disease Control and Prevention, or CDC, is part of the Department of Health and Human Services. The organization works with many officials in the field of health care to protect, preserve, and improve public health.

Chronic obstructive pulmonary disease: A chronic lung disease that can make it harder to breath. It is a progressive disease that gets worse over time. Chronic bronchitis and chronic emphysema are considered subsets of COPD. Those with this condition face a reduced life span and many side effects, including reliance on machines to ease their breathing. Smokers and all those exposed to secondhand smoke are at increased risk of COPD.

Cigarettes: Cigarettes are rolled and rounded objects that typically contain tobacco, nicotine, and other chemicals. Users may purchase pre-made cigarettes or choose to create their own. With the introduction of mechanization, it has become possible to produce them in mass quantities and make them available for consumers around the world.

Cold turkey: The act of stopping an addiction immediately and completely. Cold turkey is a method used to immediately stop using a product or substance known to be harmful. People who quit smoking cold turkey do so without outside help. Only effective for small percentage of smokers and vapers.

Electronic cigarettes: Also known as e-cigs, electronic cigarettes use a battery-operated mechanism to produce a vaporized stream that users inhale. Electronic cigarettes typically contain nicotine but need not do so.

Family Smoking Prevention and Tobacco Control Act (TCA): An Obama-era law that grants the Food and Drug Administration full authority to regulate the manufacture, marketing, and sale of all tobacco products in the United States.

Nicotine: Nicotine is a substance found in several plants including tobacco. A highly addictive chemical, nicotine is found in cigarettes and many forms of electronic cigarettes.

Nicotine replacement therapy: Nicotine replacement therapy is a form of therapy designed to help smokers quit. Users are given access to varied forms of nicotine, including gum and lozenges. Over a period of several weeks, users gradually taper down the amount of nicotine they ingest with the goal of stopping smoking altogether. When combined with other forms of therapy, Nicotine replacement therapy can be very effective.

Secondhand smoke: Secondhand smoke, also known as passive smoking, is what is produced when a smoker uses tobacco and many nicotine products. These products are known to contain thousands of potentially dangerous chemicals. Over time, bystanders who are exposed to these products can be at risk from many chronic and dangerous conditions, including heart disease, strokes, and cancer.

Social smoking: A social smoker is someone who only smokes occasionally. Many social smokers only smoke when with peers who are smoking. Studies indicate that social smoking poses many of the same risks as other kinds of smoking behaviors.

Thirdhand smoke: Thirdhand smoke is residue from smoking. Chemicals can coat a room's walls, bedding, and other soft surfaces. Tobacco and other chemicals found in smoke can emit dangerous gasses again that pose a threat to residents. All those who live with smokers or are renting or buying a home should be aware of the potential damage a previous history of smoking may pose. This is one of many reasons why smoking should be discouraged.

Tobacco: Tobacco is a plant. Grown in many parts of the world, tobacco is dried and then fermented. It is the major ingredient in tobacco products such as cigars and cigarettes.

Vaping: Vaping is the process of inhaling the aerosol of an electronic cigarette or e-cig. Vapers use a device to heat up an e-liquid. This substance is then inhaled. Vaping is often marketed as a means of quitting smoking despite studies indicating no such results. Many teens are vaping rather than using cigarettes in the belief that it is not harmful. Parents, educators, and teens should be aware that these products are dangerous and should be avoided.

Directory of Resources

BOOKS AND ARTICLES

Brandt, Allan M. *The Cigarette Century: The Rise, Fall, and Deadly Persistence of the Product That Defined America.* New York: Hachette Book Group, 2009.

Burns, Eric. *The Smoke of the Gods: A Social History of Tobacco.* New York: Temple University Press, 2006.

Gately, Iain. *Tobacco: A Cultural History of How an Exotic Plant Seduced Civilization.* New York: Grove Press, 2002.

Harrald, Chris. *The Cigarette Book: The History and Culture of Smoking.* New York: Skyhorse, 2010.

Hilts, Philip. *Smokescreen: The Truth behind the Tobacco Industry Cover-Up.* New York: Addison-Wesley, 1996.

Kluger, Richard. *Ashes to Ashes: America's Hundred-Year Cigarette War, the Public Health, and the Unabashed Triumph of Philip Morris.* New York: Alfred A. Knopf, 1996.

Nichols, Sharon L., and Thomas L. Good. *America's Teenagers—Myths and Realities: Media Images, Schooling, and the Social Costs of Careless Indifference.* Mahwah, NJ: Lawrence Erlbaum Associates Publishers, 2004.

Zegart, Dan. *Civil Warriors: The Legal Siege on the Tobacco Industry.* New York: Delta, 2001.

WEBSITES AND ORGANIZATIONS

American Lung Association: www.lung.org
Website of the American Lung Association, including information on the dangers of smoking.

Become an Ex: https://www.becomeanex.org/
Detailed assistance for those of all ages determined to be ex-smokers.

Be Tobacco Free: https://betobaccofree.hhs.gov/
Government-sponsored list of smoking-related resources.

Campaign for Tobacco Free Kids: https://www.tobaccofreekids.org/
Organized state and national antismoking campaigns kids can join.

Centers for Disease Control and Prevention (CDC): Youth Tobacco Prevention https://www.cdc.gov/tobacco/basic_information/youth/index.htm
CDC-sponsored resources devoted to teens and smoking.

My Last Dip: https://mylastdip.com/
Website designed for all those looking for help quitting smokeless tobacco.

No Smoking Room: http://nosmokingroom.org/index.html
Website for girls trying to quit smoking.

1-800-QUIT-NOW https://smokingcessationleadership.ucsf.edu/1-800-quit-now-cards
Immediate help quitting smoking from experts.

Project Prevent Youth Coalition: http://www.sosprojectprevent.com/
Teen resources devoted to lobbying against smoking in local communities and nationwide.

Smoke Free: https://smokefree.gov/
Help for those interested in quitting smoking.

Smoking Stinks: https://kidshealth.org/en/kids/smoking.html
Information and advice about smoking from pediatricians.

Still Blowing Smoke: https://stillblowingsmoke.org/
Articles on the vaping industry.

Students Working against Tobacco: http://www.swatflorida.com/
Florida government–based organization devoted to antismoking efforts.

Teen Smoke-Free: https://teen.smokefree.gov/
Government-sponsored resources for teens who want to quit smoking.

Teens against Tobacco Use: https://www.lung.org/local-content/minne sota/support-and-community/tatu.html
Peer-led antismoking campaign from the American Lung Association.

The Truth® Campaign: https://www.thetruth.com/
Nonprofit organization aiming to eliminate smoking and vaping in the United States.

Truth Initiative: https://truthinitiative.org/
America's largest nonprofit antismoking public health organization.

Youth Engagement Alliance for Tobacco Control: https://youthengage mentalliance.org/
Grassroots organization aiming to organize teens in favor of antismoking and antivaping laws.

Index

Acne, 71, 72
Addiction, xxv, xxvi, xxvii, 6, 14, 63, 64, 87, 88, 89, 90, 92, 96, 101, 105, 108
Age related macular degeneration (AMD), 54, 71
Alcohol, 15, 29, 72, 87, 88, 107–9, 122
American Academy of Pediatrics, 23
American Cancer Society, 16, 52
American Tobacco Expo, 12
Antismoking campaigns, 22, 102, 105, 112
Arthritis, 57, 58
Asia, 7, 8, 20
Asthma, xxvi, 29, 31, 54, 55, 67
Australia, 21

Bhutan, 78
Birth control, 41
Brazil, 4, 21, 22, 79
Bronchitis, xxvi, 15, 43, 72, 75, 76

Canada, 79, 80, 81
Carbon monoxide, 18, 27, 45

Cardiac arrest, 40
Centers for Disease Control and Prevention, 12, 18, 23, 50
China, 12, 19, 21, 80, 81, 82
Chronic obstructive pulmonary disease (COPD), 43, 44, 125
Cigarettes, xxv, xxvii, 5, 6, 7, 8, 9, 10, 16, 17, 22, 23, 25, 28, 30, 32, 33, 34, 35, 39, 45, 46, 48, 51, 66, 67, 68, 69, 71, 72, 74, 76, 77, 78, 80, 81, 83, 84, 85, 88, 89, 91, 92, 99, 106, 109
Cleft palate, 55, 61
Clove cigarettes, 8–9
Cocaine, 6, 13, 24, 62–63, 88, 110
Columbia University, 62

Deeming Rule, 25
Dementia, 48, 55
Diabetes, 55, 56, 70, 72, 91, 108
Dopamine, 6, 34, 36, 40, 88, 89

Ectopic pregnancy, 56, 60
Esophagus, 18, 26, 54, 61, 65
Europe, 3, 5, 8, 12, 21, 73, 74, 78, 80

Food and Drug Administration, 10, 11, 13, 69, 77, 96, 97

Germany, 21, 60, 82
Glaucoma, 54, 71

Harvard, 14
Heroin, 6, 13, 24, 62, 63, 110
HIV, 20, 72
Hon Lik, 12
Hookahs, 8

India, 4, 21, 80, 82
Indonesia, 8, 19, 21, 80, 82

Japan, 21, 82
Johns Hopkins University, 110

Kahn, Harold, 35
Kennedy, John Fitzgerald, 75

Leukemia, 16, 17, 28, 53, 60
Light smoking, xxvi, 68–69, 71, 91, 92
Lung cancer, 28, 36, 42, 43, 49–51, 52, 59, 67, 69, 72, 75, 102, 111
Lungs, 7, 14, 15, 16, 17, 18, 26, 27, 30, 31, 40–44, 46, 51, 54, 58, 66, 67, 68, 69, 71
Lupus, 57

Mayo Clinic, 43, 108
Middle East, 8, 81
Mucus, 40, 42, 43, 54

National Cancer Institute, 66, 69, 71, 111
New Jersey, 66, 69, 71, 111
Nicotine: acid reflux, 54; addiction, 13, 15, 62–63, 87; alcohol use, 108; appetite, 36; body chemistry, 7; brain, 6, 47, 48, 52, 62, 88–89, 105; cancer, 53; cardiovascular health, children, 46; delivery systems, 10; diabetes, 56; e-cigs, 13, 70; gum, 92, 93; hearing loss, 56; heart, 45; history, 4; infertility, 56; lozenge, 92, 93; Parkinson's disease, 36; patch, 92, 94; plants, 3; poisoning, 15, 65; pregnancy, 62; premature balding, 57; quitting smoking, 88; replacement therapy, 92, 96; spray, 94; thirdhand smoking, 68; ulcerative colitis, 35; vaccines, 110

Obama, Barack, 23, 69, 77
Obesity, 91
Oxygen, 26, 27, 42, 43, 45, 61, 65

Passive smoking, 28, 29, 66
Philadelphia, 74
Pipes, 8

Quitting, 62, 66, 87–90, 92, 93, 94, 97, 98, 99, 101, 102, 103, 105, 107, 109, 110, 111, 113

Red blood cells, 26, 27

Secondhand smoking, 27–29, 66, 68, 103
Sickle cell anemia, 41
Sidestream smoke, 28, 66
SIDS, 13, 28, 67
Snuff or smokeless tobacco, 5, 8, 19, 27, 64–65, 74, 83
Social smoking, 24, 71, 74, 77, 88, 90, 91
Stanford University, 85
Strokes, 29, 33, 41, 44, 45, 48, 59, 65, 67, 69, 70, 72, 76, 91, 92, 108, 126
Surgeon general's report, 74–76
Sweden, 21, 59

Thirdhand smoking, 29–33, 66–68, 103
Tobacco: advertising, 23, 83–85; bans, 76–77; chewing tobacco,

64–66; dissolvable, 8; growing methods, 3–5; harmful substances, 18; taxes, 19, 79, 80, 84; women, 19, 22, 110–11; world regulation, 78–80
Trachea, 26, 42

United Kingdom, 21, 36, 79
United States: annual lung cancer cases, 49; different rates of smoking, 19; prohibition, 76; secondhand smoke, 29; smoking popularity WWII, 74; tobacco advertising, 83; tobacco healthcare costs, 82; Tobacco Nation, 19; tobacco taxes, 80; tobacco use decline, 18
University of Alabama at Birmingham, 51

University of California: Los Angeles, 47; San Francisco, 51, 59
University of Rochester, 15

Vaping: asthma, 54; brain effects, 48; compared to low tar cigarettes, 68–70; FDA regulations, 28; general information, 10–14; hearing loss, 56; industry regulation, 77, 80; pregnancy, 61–62; quitting side effects, 99–100
Volatile organic compounds, 15, 31

Wagner, Honus, 83
World Health Organization, 21, 78
World War II, 18, 58, 73, 84

Yale University, 36, 109, 111

About the Author

Stacy Mintzer Herlihy is a parent, writer, and health advocate from New Jersey. She is the coauthor of *Your Baby's Best Shot: Why Vaccines Are Safe and Save Lives* and the founder of New Jersey Parents for Vaccines. Her work has appeared in many publications, including *Big Apple Parents*, *Today's Parents*, *USA Today*, and the *Newark Star Ledger*.